I'D KILL FOR A COOKIE

Catherine Christie

I'D KILL FOR A COOKIE

A SIMPLE SIX-WEEK PLAN TO CONQUER STRESS EATING

Susan Mitchell, Ph.D., R.D., L.D., and
Catherine Christie, Ph.D., R.D., L.D.

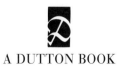

A DUTTON BOOK

NOTE TO THE READER
The ideas, procedures, and suggestions contained in this book are not intended as a substitute for consulting with your physician. All matters regarding your health require medical supervision.

DUTTON
Published by the Penguin Group
Penguin Books USA Inc., 375 Hudson Street, New York, New York 10014, U.S.A.
Penguin Books Ltd, 27 Wrights Lane, London W8 5TZ, England
Penguin Books Australia Ltd, Ringwood, Victoria, Australia
Penguin Books Canada Ltd, 10 Alcorn Avenue, Toronto, Ontario, Canada M4V 3B2
Penguin Books (N.Z.) Ltd, 182–190 Wairau Road, Auckland 10, New Zealand

Penguin Books Ltd, Registered Offices:
Harmondsworth, Middlesex, England

First published by Dutton, an imprint of Dutton Signet, a division of Penguin Books USA Inc. Distributed in Canada by McClelland & Stewart Inc.

First Printing, March, 1997
10 9 8 7 6 5 4 3

Illustrations by Melinda Kilbeck

LIBRARY OF CONGRESS CATALOGING-IN-PUBLICATION DATA:
Mitchell, Susan, Ph. D.
I'd kill for a cookie : a simple six-week plan to conquer stress eating / Susan Mitchell and Catherine Christie.
    p. cm.
Includes bibliographical references and index.
ISBN 0-525-94142-8 (alk. paper)
1. Compulsive eating—Treatment. 2. Stress management. 3. Food habits—Psychological aspects. I. Christie, Catherine. II. Title.
RC552.C65M56 1997
616.85'26—dc21   96–41985
                                                                                                      CIP

Printed in the United States of America
Set in Times Roman
Designed by Jesse Cohen

This book is printed on acid-free paper. ∞

To my mother and father, Dorothy and Lawson Mitchell, who gave me their unconditional love and encouragement to reach for my dreams.

To my brothers, Ross and Dudley, whose commitment to family will never be forgotten.

To my husband, Charlie, who renews me daily with love and joy.

—Dr. Susan Mitchell

To my husband, Leo, without whose love and support I would definitely kill for a cookie.

To my parents, Joseph and Virginia Wilcox, and my brother, Ben, who model the values and goals that I strive for each day.

To my daughter, Tara, who helps keep me young.

—Dr. Cathy Christie

ACKNOWLEDGMENTS

We would especially like to thank Jamie Pope, M.S., R.D., and Debra Waterhouse, M.P.H., R.D., two successful authors who were willing to share their experience and expertise unselfishly.

Our sincere appreciation to our agent, Judith Riven, who was willing to guide us expertly through this venture. Without her commitment to us, this book would not have become a reality.

To Debra Fulghum Bruce: It is impossible to describe how much your creative writing ability, positive attitude, support, and consistent encouragement have meant to us along the way. We are extremely grateful for the privilege of working with you.

To Deborah Brody, our editor: Your belief in *I'd Kill for a Cookie* from the beginning inspired us as we turned ideas into a completed manuscript. We are so proud to be associated with Dutton.

And to the following very special family, friends, and colleagues, thank you for being there, listening, encouraging, and believing in us:

Kay, Ben, Virginia and Elizabeth Braddock; Dorine Smith, R.D.; Marlene and Butch Stiwalt; Laura Kittleson; Ellen T. Carroll, M.S., R.D.; Debbie Hebrank, R.D.; Glenna Raidt, R.D.; Dan Raidt; Judy Cipra; Terri Langford, R.N.; Martie Salt Tucker; John Soper; Tandy Craig; Jeff Slater; Dee Tomkins; Jo Shuford Law, M.S.; and Richard Law; Patty Thomas, R.D.; Ben T. Wilcox; Buzz and Sue Crane; Leo and Theresa Christie; Carolyn and Bill Rayboun; Toni Martin, M.Ph., R.D.; Claire Lorbeer, M.S., R.D.; Alice Rhatigan, M.S., R.D.; Vilma Willard, M.S., R.D.; Lori Valencic, M.S., R.D.

We would also like to recognize the hard work and dedication of the many researchers whose quest for knowledge led to the findings reported in this book.

CONTENTS

INTRODUCTION:
HOW TO CONQUER
STRESS EATING

Would you kill for a cookie too? There are times when most everyone can identify with that feeling. When clients say to us, "You probably won't understand what I am going through, but I am completely stressed out," we do understand. We have both experienced extreme stress at different times in our lives. Cathy Christie's busy traveling and speaking schedule keeps her constantly juggling her career with family responsibilities. In the past, Cathy's response to stress was to stress-eat and gain fifteen pounds. Today, she is more likely to eat too little when under stress. Susan Mitchell has endured much personal stress in going through a divorce and losing as many family members in the last five years as most people experience losing in an entire lifetime. Her response was to stop eating and drop down to 104 pounds. At five feet six inches tall, she felt terrible.

Dr. Cathy Christie

I first became aware of the effects of stress eating during my freshman year in college. My friends and I used to joke about the weight gain we experienced as the "famous freshman ten." I was away from home for the first time, living in a dormitory with a room-mate whom I had never met before, and adjusting to the demands of a difficult college course load. Stress eating resulted in about a fifteen-pound weight gain the first semester. When I saw my parents at the semester break, I still remember my dad saying, "Catherine, what happened to your weight?" I knew that I had to make some immediate changes and began to apply what I was learning in my study of nutrition.

More recently, I have been confronted with stress eating again. I teach seminars on nutrition for health professionals across the nation, requiring travel away from my home three days each week. In addition to the pressure of preparing and presenting the seminars, the amount of travel itself is very stressful. Not only do I have to go to the next site on schedule, but I have to plan on eating out every meal. For those of you who travel or eat out frequently, you know the food available often leaves much to be desired from a health standpoint. I recall one instance after giving a six-hour seminar when I arrived at the airport to find that my flight was canceled and it was the last flight of the night. I had to rent a car and drive five hours to the next day's seminar and eat on the way—exhausted, hungry, stressed, and anx-ious, with no good food options.

Putting all of my knowledge about stress and its effects on eating into practice, I have designed an eating plan that keeps me prepared for the demands of a rigorous travel schedule. It includes carrying bottled water with me, ordering vegetarian meals on airplanes and often in hotel restaurants, and making sure I eat frequently on the road to keep up my energy level.

I speak from professional and personal experience that the EAT Plan we present in this book really does work. It has helped me and hundreds of clients prioritize what is important in our daily schedules and stop stress eating in its tracks.

DR. SUSAN MITCHELL

Perhaps my stress experience is a bit more traumatic than Cathy's, but I, too, am no stranger to the ravages of tremendous, ongoing stress. I had to find realistic and successful ways to combat stress and stress eating as I faced major surgery, divorce, and the deaths of my parents and a brother.

During this four-year period, I felt that I looked much older than my age. Because my stomach always felt so uneasy and I couldn't eat, I lost a lot of weight. At five six, weighing 104 pounds, I knew this sick feeling inside could not continue or my health would be destroyed. I needed to pull information from my education and professional experience and practice positive ways to lower my stress level and allow me to deal with the situations at hand.

I have since realized that stress will never go away completely for any of us, and I have used our stress-less strategies to deal with the pressures that confront me. My winning stress-less strategy is to graze (eat small, healthful meals frequently) and exercise consistently. I am now back to a healthy weight, am calmer, and can think more clearly, especially when faced with tough decisions.

WE'VE BEEN THERE, AND WE'VE FOUND THE ANSWERS!

The reality is that all of us will face different situations in our lives, some more difficult and painful than others. But one thing we know for sure is that the way you eat and take care of yourself makes a profound difference in the way you cope with stress every day of your life. Not only do we know from our professional training that the six-week EAT Plan works, but we both speak with the voice of having been there. In addition, as part of our research for this book, we surveyed over 1,000 adults on the topic of stress eating. What they told us confirmed what we experienced for ourselves and observed with our clients. For example, chocolate was clearly the most commonly eaten food in times of stress—but you probably already knew that. What you may not have known is that you are not alone as a stress eater. We found that two out of every three people stress-eat, most overeating and some undereating. So you see, through our work with clients and in our search for workable techniques to make the most of personal stress, we realized an unmet need in our society: specific methods that really work to conquer stress eating.

Psychologists and psychiatrists tell us that stress is one of the most pervasive battles in our society today. Perhaps you know personally that stress can play havoc with your energy level and performance, not to mention its adverse effects on your body and weight. The problem arises when everyday stress becomes *distress* or *harmful* because there are too many demands to handle and no outlet for relief.

While most people know what daily situations cause them stress, few truly understand how to make it work for them—until now. We have found, however, that if you are willing to look at your life, evaluate those pressure situations and your personal response, and then assess your nutrition and exercise habits, you *can* overcome stress and the resulting stress eating just as we have.

STRESS IS *NOT* GOING AWAY

Often it isn't the event itself that causes stress, but our *perception* of it. For example, the findings in studies of recent catastrophes show that as long as six years after a significant event, many people still experienced stress stemming from it. Their immunity was suppressed and their blood pressure was still elevated, while others recovered after just a few days. Why? Because some people have learned to view stress positively and can cope with uncomfortable situations better than others.

Learning to view stress as a positive life interruption and learning to change eating and exercise behaviors to deal with this will not be easy. It is going to take some lifestyle and emotional housekeeping on your part. But as you start the EAT Plan and practice the six stress-less strategies, not only are you going to look and feel better, you will also have the energy and skills to deal with the unending stresses of daily life, whether minor or monumental.

Our book has two major purposes:

- To provide a deeper understanding of how stress affects you personally—your health, your motivation and productivity, and your moods
- To provide the solution to the growing prevalence of stress eating with an innovative but easy-to-understand program we call the EAT Plan

The EAT Plan is your Energy-Action Team. The team approach will work with your strengths and fill in where problems exist so you can make the stress in your life work *with* you instead of against you.

Your Energy-Action Team consists of six stress-less strategies. As you work through your stress-less strategies, you will learn to:

1. Eat to combat stress and boost immunity;
2. Eat to enhance your mood;
3. Move to create happy hormones;
4. Plan your time and prioritize;
5. Revamp your pantry; and
6. Hit the road running.

You may say, "That's fine, but how can the EAT Plan really affect my eating habits? I've tried to control them, but no diet has worked so far."

We have discovered that the best way to conquer stress eating and gain control of your weight is to *quit dieting and start eating*. The EAT Plan will show you how to make this "dinosaur dieting" extinct while eating *more frequently* to boost your metabolism and productivity. That's right. Our six stress-less strategies will allow you to eat mini-meals throughout the day while establishing a program to alleviate the tension and anxiety caused by stress.

Recent research has found that people who eat two meals or less during the day have a slower metabolic rate (the speed at which your body burns calories, and the rate that we all want to go faster) than those who eat three or more times a day. We're going to teach you how to manage your weight and stress response by eating food and letting it work for you.

You may also ask, "But what about exercise? Isn't that important for controlling one's weight and stress? I could start an exercise program—if I had some energy."

Most clients agree that they, too, do not have the energy to go and "work it out." However, "happy hormones," or the elevated endorphin levels that result from activity, will make you feel better about life. These happy hormones will increase your self-esteem and sexual desire as well as help relieve depression. The good news is that they are absolutely free. Exercise is today's legal wonder drug that improves your mood and lowers stress. In fact, studies have proven that aerobic activity can reduce anxiety, tension, and stress, and it can increase vigor and promote clear thinking.

We know that you are busy (along with being stressed out), but we will motivate you to begin an activity and exercise regimen that you can do at home or even on the job. The EAT Plan will help

- Alleviate your feeling of unending stress and the resulting physical symptoms
- Stop the excessive cravings that are making you lose control of your eating habits and weight
- Energize you so that you are more productive at work, home, and play
- Relax you as you learn to turn off that fight-or-flight response

- Make you the "master" of your temperament as an Active Mood Manager

WORK WITH YOUR BODY'S RHYTHM

As you learn to manage your moods, we will help you discover the secret of your personal circadian rhythm. Circadian rhythms are separate, individually synchronized internal rhythms that affect our daily sleep cycles, performance and alertness, moods, and even gastrointestinal function.

Understanding whether you are an early bird or a night owl is vital in planning your day and your meals. For example, if you are an early bird who eats nothing but serotonin-boosting carbohydrates all afternoon and evening, you are setting yourself up for problems as you complete your late-day tasks in a nonproductive manner. We will show you how choosing high-protein foods at midafternoon and evening will enable you to recharge, think more clearly, and boost your energy level. On the other hand, that night owl who blindly stumbles out of bed just in time for the 8:00 A.M. business meeting and grabs a doughnut and glass of juice on the way to the office will also lose productivity and thinking power. If you are a night owl, we will show how choosing a breakfast high in brain-boosting protein, such as an egg sandwich or piece of leftover pizza, will perk you up and increase your alertness.

CONTROL YOUR WEIGHT

In our practice, we have found that clients with all types of stress who start the EAT Plan and maintain a regular exercise program are able to see and feel improvement in all areas of their lives, including weight management. Our diverse clients have brought to our attention stress-eating scenarios ranging from the corporate executive who never eats a meal until he gets home in the evening but survives the day with black coffee, calorie-laden sweet rolls, and a package of

Tums in his briefcase, to the accountant who cannot control her weight or her stress level because she sits all day at a computer while snacking too much and exercising too little.

They both complain of having no energy and know that their health is suffering, but, like so many people short on time and long on stress, they need to learn how to cope effectively.

In today's world, we know that successful people do more with less and do it better; increased productivity is the name of the game, whether you manage a business or a home. And this success theory applies to all areas of your life as you learn to set daily priorities; plan your meals and snacks for a positive food-mood connection; engage in a regular fitness program of activity and exercise; practice meditation, visualization, or other relaxation techniques throughout the day; learn to incorporate nutritious foods with healing phytochemicals and antioxidants into your meal plan; and eat well when you are away from home.

RELAXATION IS REJUVENATING

Relaxation techniques can trigger the relaxation response—a physiological state characterized by a feeling of warmth and quiet mental alertness. This is the opposite of the fight-or-flight response. Once you learn how to use the relaxation response taught in the EAT Plan, blood flow to the brain increases and brain waves shift from an alert, beta rhythm to a relaxed, alpha rhythm. Practiced regularly, relaxation techniques can counteract the debilitating effects of stress. When an Oregon nursing professor taught relaxation techniques to thirty-eight nursing students, she found that they scored substantially lower on a scale rating stress, anxiety, and depression after only three weeks. A group of students who received no training scored higher on this scale over the same period.

THE EAT PLAN HAS HELPED THOUSANDS

Do these strategies work for everyone? While we cannot guarantee that the EAT Plan will work for every person who picks up this book, we do know that these strategies have worked in our personal lives and for thousands of our busiest clients as they made a commitment to learn the plan and incorporate the stress-less strategies into their daily lives.

The key ingredient in ending stress eating is *you*. You can start right now to take control of your life and make stress work *for* you by learning from those who have been there and who are winning the fight with stress eating.

In this book we provide you with practical tools and successful techniques for resolving stress eating and regaining control of your life. With these tools, you can discover the key stressors in your life and learn to deal with them in a positive manner that will benefit your health, your relationships, and your career.

Now let's get started!

chapter 1

────── ◦ ──────

ALL STRESSED UP AND
NO PLACE TO GO

The feeling crashes over you like a surging ocean wave: Your heart rate goes into high gear, your head pounds, and you feel nervous and short of breath. What could be wrong? In most cases, this reaction is not life-threatening but, rather, a common one to compounded daily stress and anxiety.

Stress. We all live with it from day to day, and you'd have to agree that just hearing the word can make you cringe. Whether it is a confrontation with your boss, a ranting and raving argument with your teenager, or living with chronic pain, stress is here to stay. When someone mentions stress, don't you immediately think about everything you don't have time to do? Sometimes it seems your ever-increasing list of things to do can leave you feeling totally undone. All you know is that the demands of your day greatly overshadow the number of hours you have available, and you never have time for yourself.

A recent poll by the Gallup Organization revealed that for more than half of those age thirty-five to fifty-four stress is a familiar part of their daily lives. Job and financial problems were the leading stressors. For many career people, even when they leave work for the day, any downtime is spent negotiating deals with clients on cellular phones or answering faxes and E-mail at home. No matter if you are dealing with downsizing, mergers and layoffs, or kids, car pools, and housework, it isn't news that many Americans today work twenty-four hours a day, seven days a week—even when they are not supposed to be "at work."

How often do you feel stressed? One recent survey found that 16 percent of those questioned felt stressed "all the time" and could not seem to relax, not even for a minute, while 52 percent of those questioned felt stressed "most of the time." Every week, some 95 million Americans suffer a stress-related problem and take medication for their aches and pains. Whether it stems from phones ringing off the hook, being bombarded with news of crime and violence around the world, or living with a colicky baby that won't stop crying, stress inundates the body with stress hormones that don't quit. It also creates a host of unpleasant physical symptoms. You may suffer from an increased number of stress-related physical complaints such as headache, backache, edginess, sweaty hands, difficulty in concentrating, or upset stomach. Or you may react to stress as two out of every three people do, with stress eating. This means eating loads of extra calories, from candy to tortilla chips, or practically starving yourself by drinking diet sodas and coffee all day and eating little else.

Mona, a busy high school principal and mother of three, knows all about reacting to daily stress with overeating. She tells of feeling as if she has an internal switch that immediately turns on her appetite when she feels overwhelmed. "When I get to school and see hundreds of teens push through the crowded hallways, I immediately head to the teachers' lounge for coffee and doughnuts. It's an automatic response that I cannot seem to control, and I'm paying for it with extra weight."

For others, like Jeff, the switch turns off any signs of an appetite. When Jeff's youngest child was put in the hospital for a week of medical tests, he described feeling like there was a sponge in his throat. "The thought of food repulsed me, so I lived on diet colas and crackers the entire time," Jeff said.

What happens when you feel stress? Most people tell of feeling angry, burned out, powerless, or sad, and react to these emotions in a destructive manner—with unhealthy eating habits. In fact, researchers have found that during times of stress, people are either eaters like Mona or noneaters like Jeff; half of men eat more and half of men eat less, while two-thirds of women eat more and one-third eat less.

THE *SOUND OF MUSIC* SYNDROME

Time and time again, our clients seek assistance with weight control. Upon counseling them, we realize that they first need help controlling the stress in their lives. Better still, realizing that stress is here to stay, they need help in making the stress in their lives work *for* them instead of *against* them. Many tell of coping with stress with what we call the "Sound of Music Syndrome." This means eating a few of their favorite things, such as brownies, cookies, french fries, and sodas. But the agonizing truth is that after a fat-sugar binge, the stress is still there and so is the resulting unwanted weight gain.

Don't give up just yet. If you are overdosing on stress, we'll show you how to find relief. From our experience with clients, we have found that once you understand the specific stressors in your life, you can learn creative changes to make life's stressors work for you. You can change your food-reaction to stress and its effect on your life and your weight no matter what your circumstances.

EVERYONE HAS STRESS

Whatever stress you face in life, the comforting news is that you are not alone. Millions of people today feel all stressed up with no place to go. The problem with feeling stressed day after day is that you will ultimately face burnout, and as most of us know, burnout virtually means "worn out." Perhaps you are only partially there and suffer from brownout, but the results will ultimately be the same. The following checklist may help you determine how the stress of daily living is affecting you.

STRESS SYMPTOM INVENTORY

Think back over the past few weeks. Rate the given stress symptoms according to their frequency using the following scale:

3 = Daily

2 = Frequently

1 = Rarely

0 = Never

_____   1. I feel tired or run down.

_____   2. I get angry or frustrated easily.

_____   3. I have lost interest in my work.

_____   4. Stress bothers me more now than before.

_____   5. I get headaches or stomachaches regularly.

_____   6. I have trouble sleeping.

_____   7. I feel depressed or unhappy frequently.

_____   8. I have lost my sense of humor.

_____   9. I have become more rigid and critical.

_____ 10. I feel overwhelmed or overworked.

_____ 11. I frequently use mood-altering drugs or alcohol.

_____ 12. I clench my jaws while sleeping.

_____ 13. I have lost or gained weight recently.

Now total up your points and use the following scale to see how you scored:

27–39: Red alert! Your score indicates burnout, but there is hope. As you read this book, you can identify your stressors and learn stress-less strategies, including relaxation techniques to get out of the danger range.

14–26: Warning, warning: Your score indicates brownout. While you are not totally stressed, you are rapidly heading in that direction so don't put this book down yet. Learn the warning signs and stress-less strategies to protect yourself.

0–13: Terrific. Today stress is working for you. To stay away from the stress-eating trap, keep reading for some easy-to-follow tips to keep you on track.

OUR STRESS-LESS STRATEGIES REALLY WORK

Whether your stress test indicated brownout or burnout, this book will teach you our innovative EAT Plan, which will allow you to turn stress in your favor before it manages you and takes its toll on your mental, emotional, and physical well-being. But let's first explain why we all react to stress in our daily lives.

WHAT'S YOUR REACTION?

Our clients tell us and we know ourselves about all kinds of unhealthy or uncomfortable reactions to stress, from clenched jaws, headaches, and insomnia to lack of energy, weight gain, and weight loss. Some clients, like Jack, an accountant and single parent, describe losing their sense of humor. "I become rigid and unyielding during tax season," Jack told us. "You can ask my kids; until midnight on April fifteenth, I'm no fun to be around." Carolyn, a busy mother and teacher, asked us if the word *relaxation* had its derivative from a foreign language. "It sure isn't in my vocabulary," she said. Then we have those clients like Rob, a recently divorced police officer who doesn't recognize the symptoms of too much stress, yet wonders why he cannot stop gaining weight. "I'm being honest when I tell you that I only eat one meal when I come home from work," Rob told us, "but why do I keep gaining weight?" (Rob forgot to mention that his one meal lasted from 6:00 P.M. until he went to bed.)

How about you? Have you counted the many hats you wear every day? Perhaps you are juggling an upwardly mobile career while trying to be a "super" parent and keep your marriage together, and you want to do it all. Well, take heart, you are not alone. Most of us are in the same boat with too many demands on our time, even when we enjoy them, yet they all add up to one key word called *stress*.

UNDERSTANDING STRESS

To help you understand how stress affects your eating habits, let's first analyze what constitutes stress. Simply stated, stress describes the many demands and pressures that all people experience to some degree each day. These demands may be physical, mental, emotional, or even chemical in nature. The word *stress* includes both the stressful situation, known as the stressor, and the symptoms you experience under stress, your stress response.

Just about anything you encounter can cause stress. Usually it is not life's emergencies or disasters that trigger the majority of stress reactions, but more often it is the persistent interruptions, hassles, and struggles you face every day. Whether you are confronted with financial or health problems, waiting in long lines of traffic each evening, or raising active children, all can add up to overwhelming stress, resulting in stress eating.

THE EAT PLAN SURVEY RESULTS

We found in our survey of more than 1,000 adults that 79 percent of women and 69 percent of men reported stress eating. The most common food category was sweets, and chocolate was by far the most frequent sweet eaten. The second most common food category for stress eating was salty foods, with potato chips topping the list. Women were most likely to stress-eat when anxious, bored, or sad, while men were most likely to stress-eat when bored or lonely. Both sexes reported that their largest meal was dinner, and when breakfast was eaten, the most common foods chosen were cereal, toast, and fruit. When breakfast was skipped, the most common reason was lack of time.

Both men and women face stress in their lives, but studies show that women are more likely to report feeling at least a moderate amount of stress and feeling that this stress has affected their health. We have found that women are also more likely to seek professional help for stress-related problems, while men are less likely to reveal their concerns about stress.

Whether male or female, whenever we encounter stress it requires us to change or adapt in some fashion; it interrupts our daily schedule. For example, being stuck in slow-moving traffic during rush hour requires that we change our expectations about arriving at our destination at an expected time, and for most of us, having to change our plans makes us tense and irritable. Similarly, the stress of going through a critical job interview requires that we do our best to maintain a relaxed, self-assured, and confident approach and make a good impression. And what parent hasn't experienced the stress of trying to entertain energetic children on long summer days while maintaining his or her sanity? Usually this requires flexibility, calmness, and control that few of us feel. As contradictory as it may seem, trying to stay relaxed in moments of uncertainty creates great stress for most of us.

STRESS CAUSES ILLNESS

Clearly, research indicates that stress is not only uncomfortable but that long-term stress leads to health problems. The Department of Health and Human Services reports that 43 percent of adults suffer adverse health effects from stress. It is also estimates that at least 85 percent of all workplace accidents could be caused by difficulties employees face in coping with emotional distress. Reports vary, but emotional stress has been implicated in more than 50 percent of all visits to the hospital, and stress has been linked to increased risk of the following diseases:

High blood pressure	Cancer
Stroke	Allergies, asthma, and hay fever
Heart disease	Rheumatoid arthritis
Ulcers	Backaches
Migraine headaches	TMJ (temporomandibular joint
Tension headaches	syndrome)

These stress-induced illnesses add up to $30 billion a year in medical bills and disability payments in our country. And American businesses lose an estimated $150 billion each year due to employee stress-related problems. According to a survey conducted by CCH Inc. in 1994, these unscheduled stress-related absences from work can cost a company as much as $750 per employee absence. All of us know the feeling of someone being absent from work in a downsizing environment. You are already faced with "do more with less, and do it better." Then someone calls in sick and you must pick up the slack. And it's not just at work. What do you do when your three-year-old wakes up with chicken pox and there's no sitter in sight, yet you have a doctor's appointment you just can't miss? Watch out, here it comes—more stress.

STRESS PUTS YOU AT RISK

Because stress contributes to increased blood pressure and cholesterol, it is not surprising that it is associated with a greater risk of stroke and heart disease. The reason for this is that stress pumps you up, causing an adrenaline release, which sets up a whole cascade of reactions, including increased heart rate and blood pressure. Stress has also been associated with increased production of cholesterol in the liver. One study examined the serum cholesterol levels of male tax accountants during tax season and during a less stressful time frame. When the variables of eating erratically and exercising less due to the increased work load were controlled, stress accounted for a 10 percent increase in serum cholesterol during the stressful tax season.

Women also increase their cholesterol production when stressed, but only about half as much, accounting for a rise during times of stress of about 5 percent. What may come as a surprise, however, is that the effects of stress on the immune system limit its ability to fight allergies, asthma, arthritis, and even cancer. Stress also affects muscle tension that is associated with headaches, backaches, and TMJ.

Hans Selye, an endocrinologist and biologist, was one of the first people to write about stress and its effects on our bodies, saying that stress is "the nonspecific response of the body to any demand." In his book *Stress Without Distress*, he describes the physiological response to stressors in three stages known as the General Adaptation Syndrome (GAS).

ALARM REACTION STAGE

When we are exposed to a situation perceived as threatening, our bodies prepare for confrontation. The response is physical and is controlled by our hormones and nervous system and is known as the fight-or-flight response: We are prepared to fight or flee our stressor. Even though we do not live in the age of fighting wild animals anymore, those wild animals still exist in such forms as traffic jams, long lines, and disputes with our boss or family. When confronted with a stressful situation such as a canceled flight or a sick child, the body produces adrenaline. The release of adrenaline is like sending a thousand telegrams to different parts of the body at once.

Figure1.1

ALARM REACTION STAGE

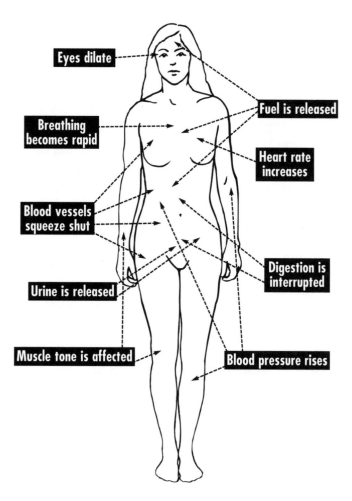

Eyes dilate

Fuel is released

Breathing becomes rapid

Heart rate increases

Blood vessels squeeze shut

Digestion is interrupted

Urine is released

Muscle tone is affected

Blood pressure rises

These telegrams prepare the body to deal with the stress, whether positive or negative (see Figure 1.1).

Blood Vessels: The vessels in the outer body squeeze shut to force blood into the vital organs such as the liver, kidneys, brain, and major muscles.

Blood Pressure: As more blood flows into the heart, blood pressure increases to circulate blood to these same major organs.

Heart Rate: Heart rate also rises to try to compensate for the increased blood pressure.

Fuel Release: In the liver, stored carbohydrate is converted to glucose (blood sugar) to provide a fuel source for the organs that need it, particularly the brain and the nervous system.

Digestion: This process is interrupted; why digest food when there is imminent danger?

Frequency of Urination: The bladder contracts and urine is released more easily so accidents can happen.

Lungs: The exchange of oxygen and carbon dioxide is enhanced when we breathe more rapidly. Therefore, more oxygen is available for the increased metabolic rate caused by the stress reaction.

Eyes: The pupils of the eyes dilate to allow adjustment to dim light. This is thought to be a response to prepare for fighting.

Muscle Tone: The tone of muscles is affected so that shaking or trembling is a common reaction to fear and to chronic emotional stress.

When the alarm stage repeatedly occurs, stress manifests itself in disrupting the body.

Figure 1.2

EFFECTS OF PROLONGED ALARM
REACTION STAGE

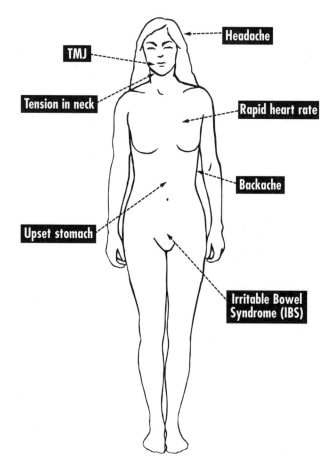

TMJ

Headache

Tension in neck

Rapid heart rate

Backache

Upset stomach

Irritable Bowel
Syndrome (IBS)

RESISTANCE STAGE

The second stage in our stress response is the body's attempt to reestablish a more normal level of functioning known as homeostasis. Typically, your headaches and upset stomachs occur in

Figure 1.3

RESISTANCE STAGE

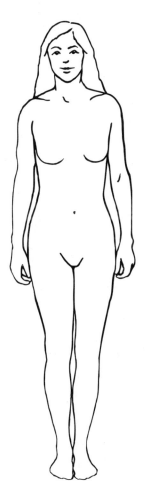

the alarm phase of stress, and your body is trying to resist these negative changes, calm the storms, and return to a more balanced pattern.

EXHAUSTION STAGE

These symptoms cannot go on forever. Ultimately, the result of undergoing a period of intensified stress is exhaustion, that feeling of being tired, stressed, and strained.

Figure 1.4

EXHAUSTION STAGE

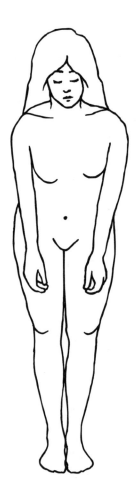

STRESS CAN BE POSITIVE OR NEGATIVE

Whether stress is viewed as positive or negative, it is as real for each of us as death and taxes. The way we perceive the stress and our feelings of control over it are what create differences in our physical and emotional responses. And, interestingly, life's stressors can produce the same initial physical response of adrenaline rush whether the stress is perceived as positive or negative. For example, public speaking may be a positive experience for some people but a very negative one for others. Or buying a home may be exciting for one person but very stressful for someone else.

EUSTRESS

Eustress, or positive stress, still signals the fight-or-flight response, which gives us the energy to enjoy these events. Positive stressors have been linked with increasing productivity, happiness, or longevity. The response to positive stressors does not advance to the third stage of the three-part GAS model, where health problems can occur.

POSITIVE STRESSORS	
Getting married	Entertaining
A new job	Shopping for clothes
Having a baby	Celebrating the holidays
Making new friends	Graduating from school
Signing a contract	Going on a vacation
Buying a house	

DISTRESS

Distress is the term for the negative side of stressors. These stressors cause the full-blown stress response and if continuous, lead to loss of productivity, health problems, and exhaustion.

NEGATIVE STRESSORS	
Chronic pain	Loss of income
Death of a loved one	Unexpected bills
Loneliness	Family problems
Fear	Unhappy career
Illness	Long-term caregiving
Losing a job	Marital problems

STRESS TRIGGERS PHYSICAL AND EMOTIONAL RESPONSES

People all respond differently to stress. Whatever the stressful situation is, from daily deadlines to rush-hour traffic to coping with your live-in mother-in-law or even to the sudden illness of a loved one, the physical response still occurs. Although this response can vary in intensity, the physical symptoms characteristic for one person will predictably happen again and again during "tense" moments.

Common Stress Reactions

Anger	IBS (irritable bowel
Anxiety	syndrome)
Apathy	Impotence
Back pain	Inability to relax
Chest pain or tightness	at night
Colitis	Inability to concentrate
Depression	Irregular menstrual periods
Headaches (including	Jaw pain
migraine and tension	Loss of sexual function
headaches)	Loss of sexual desire
Heart palpitations	Mood swings
Hives	Moodiness

Common Stress Reactions

Neck pain	Short temper
No energy	Short-term memory loss
Rapid pulse	Weight loss
Rashes	Weight gain

STRESS AND YOUR IMMUNE SYSTEM

In addition to affecting these physical symptoms, stress has also been associated with changes in our bodies at a cellular level; changes we don't even feel or see occuring daily. These changes affect our bodies' ability to respond to infection and eventually may influence our risk of illness. In short, our immune system becomes less effective. Stress-induced immune suppression has been demonstrated in situations such as adverse life events, psychological stress, and depression. And these situations are associated with the development and the course of many human diseases. One good example is the death of a spouse. Extensive studies show that this trauma is often associated with an elevated mortality rate for the survivor, particularly in the early periods after the loss. Another example is the relationship between psychological stress and the increased risk of colds. When subjects were given nasal drops containing one of five cold viruses, colds and cold symptoms increased with the amount of psychological stress. Most of us have felt that we are more vulnerable to colds when under stress, and this study supports that belief. Researchers have demonstrated decreases in cellular immune function and antibody response with stress.

When we analyze the influence of food on immune function, the new research linking antioxidants and phytochemicals to disease prevention stands out. The antioxidants act as part of the body's cell defense system. This defense is due to the antioxidant's destruction of free radicals, unstable enemies that cause cell damage. Our body cells are continually exposed to free radicals, and this exposure contributes to the development of diseases such as cancer, heart disease, and cataracts. The most powerful of the antioxidants may be vitamin C, which is found in most fruits and vegetables. Revealing studies show that this vitamin can possibly lower blood pressure, raise the levels of HDLs (good cholesterol), and decrease LDLs (bad cholesterol). The antioxidants prevent the formation of free radicals, which can damage artery walls and lead to plaque buildup.

The UCLA School of Public Health recently analyzed findings from a decade-long federal health study looking at 11,000 adults. By grouping the participants according to vitamin C intake and comparing their death rates, epidemiologist James Enstrom and his colleagues found that those consuming the most vitamin C lived the longest. Men in the highest intake group (roughly 300 milligrams each day from food and supplements) suffered 41 percent fewer deaths during the study than those with the lowest intake (less than 50 milligrams a day). The difference translates into roughly six years of added life span. As a result of the recent vitamin C research, the National Institute of Health has recommended that the daily intake should be 200 milligrams rather than the RDA level of 60 milligrams.

In another study, Harvard Medical School doctors found that when men with a history of cardiac disease were given another antioxidant, beta-carotene, as a 50-milligram supplement every other day, they suffered half as many heart attacks, strokes, and deaths as those taking a placebo pill. Scientists speculate that the antioxidant helps prevent those free radicals from transforming LDLs into an even more menacing artery clogger.

Other studies show that beta-carotene may prove powerful in combating cancer as well. In countries such as Japan and Norway, where diets are rich in beta-carotene, the populations have a low incidence of lung, colon, prostate, cervical, and breast cancer. And a recent study at the University of Arizona Cancer Center found that three to six months of daily beta-carotene pills dramatically reduced precancerous mouth lesions in 70 percent of the patients. However, in a study of smokers, beta-carotene supplements were associated with an increased risk of lung cancer. Food sources of carotenoids (including beta-carotene) such as fruits and vegetables have universally produced beneficial health effects.

What about foods such as capsaicin-containing peppers? Some studies reveal that peppers temporarily raise one's metabolic rate. In addition, there is research into an entire area of phytochemicals, such as coumarins (found in limes, carrots, and oranges), in some foods that keep your blood clotting and may have an anticancer activity. Lycopenes, found in the red pigment of tomatoes and red grapefruit, may help the body resist cancer and its spread. And resveratrol, found in grapes, is thought to lower levels of harmful cholesterol (LDLs) and decrease arterial plaque.

HDLs: High-density lipoproteins called "good" cholesterol because they carry cholesterol to the liver for the body to remove

LDLs: Low-density lipoproteins called "bad" cholesterol because they carry cholesterol to the arteries, where plaque is formed

Free radicals: Unstable molecules that cause cell damage

Antioxidants: Chemicals found in fruits and vegetables that strengthen the defense of body cells, improve immunity, and reduce risk of disease such as cancer and heart disease

Phytochemicals: Naturally occurring chemicals found in plant foods that protect the body from disease

WHAT'S YOUR PERSONAL RESPONSE TO STRESS?

There is no "quick fix" for coping with stress, but you will learn how to combat the destructive effects of stress by eating to boost antioxidants and phytochemicals in Stress-Less Strategy #1. No matter what kind of stress you experience, it is important to understand that it is your particular response to stress that determines your relationship with food. And stress eating is not concerned with quality or quantity but only with eating to satisfy emotional needs. What usually happens when we are operating under stress is that the very foods we reach for are foods like candy, cake, cookies, chocolate, and ice cream, or hot dogs, and dip and chips. Not only do these foods affect our weight, they also affect our mental performance and energy level.

How does daily stress affect your eating habits? Look at the following questions to determine your personal stress-eating response.

STRESS-EATING ASSESSMENT

1. Are you too hurried or stressed to have time for breakfast?
   Y   N

2. Is caffeine the most important ingredient in your breakfast?
   Y   N

3. If you are trying to diet, do you skip or cut back on meals?
   Y   N

4. Around 3:00 P.M., do you have that no-energy feeling?
   Y   N

5. Are you starving when you arrive home at the end of the day?
   Y   N

6. Do you stand at the counter and eat anything you can find?
   Y   N

8. Is it your style to sample food while preparing it?

   Y N

9. Do your elbow and the remote control get the majority of exercise in the evening?

   Y N

10. When you go long periods of time without eating, do you become short-tempered and irritable?

    Y N

11. When you eat under stress, do you choose only treats?

    Y N

12. Do you stress-eat several times a week?

    Y N

13. Do you crave sweets several times a week?

    Y N

14. Have you gained or lost weight recently because of stress eating?

    Y N

15. When you are under stress, is chocolate the only food that really calms you down?

    Y N

If most of your answers were "yes," you are not alone. Our EAT Plan will help you to change these stress-eating patterns. You will gain more control of stress eating and your weight, and also learn to handle the intruding stressors in your life and make them work for you.

FOOD MAKES US FEEL SO GOOD

We have some clients who tell us from the start that they cope well with stress, but these people are exceptions. It is our experience that most busy people today do not know how to manage the various demands made by employers or employees, family members and friends. When you add to these demands a list of "mandatory" social engagements, community commitments, and the need for personal time, no wonder millions of people turn to food to relieve stress. When we are confronted with daily stressors, it is easy to relieve our inner tension with food. This acts as a comfort to many people.

We are sure that those of you who increase your calories under stress are eating more broccoli, carrots, and spinach, while those who decrease their eating are choosing carefully what they do eat to ensure good nutrition, right? Wrong. In reality, the opposite is true. Eating too few calories leads to lower energy, the inability to focus, and causes the body to exhaust its own resources. Likewise, eating too many calories can lead to weight gain and sluggishness.

In our years of teaching and private practice, countless examples of stress eating have been described to us by students or clients. Stories such as devouring an entire gallon of Breyers Pralines and Cream ice cream at one time or eating the sugary centers out of a whole bag of Oreo cookies are not uncommon. And just as common are those stories of people who go without a variety of healthy food for days and exist on peanut-butter crackers and cola drinks.

STOP—AND TAKE CONTROL

As stress levels in your life continue to climb, you may find yourself skipping meals, grabbing a bite to eat between meetings, then coming home at the end of the day starving when "arsenic hour" sets in. This is that time of the day when you are so hungry and tired that you find yourself reaching for and eating anything and everything just to satisfy your hunger. You may not even be aware that you're not thinking about taste, quantity, or nutrition. All you want at that moment is immediate gratification. **Stop!** We will show you that it does not have to be this way.

Maybe you have a headache right now while reading this book, and if we were to ask when was the last time you had a real meal, you could not remember. Yet you could tell us exactly how many cups of coffee, how many diet sodas, and how much snack food you have eaten for days on end. **Stop!** The stress-less strategies in our EAT Plan will help you halt this behavior easily.

Perhaps you are constantly bouncing back and forth between overeating and dieting in a vain attempt to lose weight and deal with your stress. You follow every new diet that comes along, only to find that when you do lose the weight, you gain it back again, plus a few more pounds. (This is called the yo-yo syndrome.) **Stop!** We can help you get back in control of your weight.

Or suppose you are handling stress and food just fine until you sit down to watch television after a tiring day. The enticing commercial for Snickers gooey candy bars comes on, and you find yourself feeling out of control; you can't live without having them. You know that you are not hungry, but you must have some. **Stop!** Again, you are not alone and can learn how to manage food cravings such as this.

STRESS LEADS TO OVEREATING

When we met Karen, she had gained fifteen pounds from stress eating. Karen was a young professional in her early thirties, whose weight gain occurred after moving to a new state and making a career change. She became very distressed while trying to meet strict deadlines and began to binge-eat during evenings at home.

Karen came to us because she had no energy, felt guilty for binge eating, and appeared depressed. She was also seeing a therapist to deal with her depression. After instituting the stress-less strategies, Karen was able to lose weight gradually and had lost about ten of her fifteen extra pounds in a three-month time frame. The real benefit she found was that no longer did she feel the need to binge on sweet foods at night, and she felt more in control of her eating. Karen told us she was more energetic and positive about her future, too.

Just a few months after Karen had started her new career, her job was eliminated. For most of us that would be a major stressor. But Karen called to say she was relocating to another state and felt confident that even with this added stress of losing her job, she would not give in to her old eating habits.

Yes, stress makes us feel out of control and can make us do things we would not do under normal relaxed circumstances—most importantly, eat. But we have some clients who react in quite the opposite way to stress, by *not* eating.

SOME QUIT EATING ALTOGETHER

One such client was Mary Ellen, an exceptionally beautiful and successful model who never had to worry about her weight. "I've weighed the same, one hundred and twenty-two pounds, since eighth grade," she told us, "until my mother became ill."

She told us of being very close to her mother as the only child, and when her mother was diagnosed with Alzheimer's disease, Mary Ellen chose to move in with her as the caregiver during her last days. Over a period of nine months until her mother's death, Mary Ellen virtually quit eating, except for cookies and a hamburger each day. She went from 122 pounds to her all-time low of 106 pounds, and she is five feet nine inches tall. You can imagine how gaunt and thin she looked. But more important than how she looked, when she came to us Mary Ellen felt horrible. She had no energy or enthusiasm for life and was even beginning to lose some of her hair. Her cheeks were sunken, and we even questioned if she wasn't the one who was ill.

Her health turned around through implementing some of our stress-less strategies, and Mary Ellen was able to take control again. While she still had to deal with the sadness of losing a parent, she committed herself to eating differently. She even kept a diary of her feelings and what she ate each day to make sure she was getting the food her body needed.

Five months later, Mary Ellen had returned to her ideal weight of 122 pounds and was modeling again. Not only did the stress-less strategies give her control of her health, but she felt a renewed enthusiasm for life and was ready to handle life's interruptions.

STRESS IS HERE TO STAY

We wish we could tell you that your stress is going to be eliminated, but by now it is probably no news to you that stress is here to stay. Life's stressors are going to interrupt you today, tomorrow, and for years to come. Some of you may even think, So what's the use of trying to cope if stress is certain in life?

While you have no control over life's stressors, there are some things you do have control over. One of the most effective ways to cope with stress is to change the way you treat yourself, including your food choices and eating style, your daily commitments, your exercise and activity level, and the way you spend any "downtime."

OUR EAT PLAN IS THE KEY

So is there an answer to coping with the ravages of daily stress? Definitely! The answer lies with the EAT Plan—your Energy-Action Team. The EAT Plan is specifically designed to help you understand the stressors in your life, focus on how you react to these stressful situations, and apply its six proven strategies to conquer stress eating. We know that with the EAT Plan, you will not only feel energized, but you will also look great and be more productive.

This book will help you to identify your stressors and evaluate them as either positive or negative. Then you can prioritize the stressors that cause you the most problems and decide which ones can be eliminated (such as saying no to someone who infringes on personal time), modified (such as avoiding traffic during rushed times), or managed (such as your mother-in-law who lives with you).

And let's not forget to mention that once you have identified and organized your stressful situations, you will discover our six easy-to-understand and practical stress-less strategies to turn your personal stressors into winning scenarios. You will learn to harness the abundant energy involved with stress and make it work for you as you learn how to include the EAT Plan in your lifestyle.

In short, you don't have to feel all stressed up with no place to go any longer. We believe that you *do* have someplace to go, and we're going to take you there.

chapter 2

GIVE ME SOME CHOCOLATE, PLEASE

"Sugar. It has such a hold on me." Barbara patted her hips while lamenting her recent weight gain of eleven pounds. "Honestly, each morning I feel so strong and tell myself that today I will be good; I will be in control and not give in to my cravings. But by three each afternoon when clients are lined up outside my door and my phone won't quit ringing, sugar seems to call my name."

The attractive professional woman lowered her eyes and in a hushed voice whispered, "When I've had a really bad day, I've been known to rummage through my partner's desk in search of M and Ms."

We envisioned this sophisticated forty-year-old mortgage banker secretly delving into never-never land in search of chocolate. But Barbara is not alone. Many clients have expressed similar concerns regarding uncontrollable cravings, especially during times of exceptional stress or turmoil. A new mother of twins told of hiding in the shower stall while she ate ranch-flavored Pringle's for breakfast each morning. "I just knew my husband would think I had fallen off the deep end if he saw me," she said, "but I had to have them."

Other clients have expressed similar food cravings, asking questions such as:

> Why do I have this uncontrollable urge to eat anything chocolate right before my period?
>
> Why do I have to have pepperoni pizza every Friday night?
>
> Why do I have a sudden urge for a nutty caramel candy bar every day when I pick up my sons from elementary school?
>
> Why do I need dessert after I do the dishes each night?
>
> Why do potato chips taste so good when I'm edgy?
>
> Why can't I go to sleep at night without a dish of chocolate ice cream?
>
> I hate popcorn, so why do I have to have it at the movie theater?
>
> Why can't I control my cravings?
>
> Tell me, is there something wrong with me?

Perhaps a most interesting craving concern came from Lori, a young middle-school teacher, who asked, "Why do I crave puréed apricot baby food for breakfast during the first month of school? The thought of it makes me sick any other time of the year."

Wow! Puréed apricot baby food? Theoretically we could not tell Lori exactly why she had that particular craving. However, we've heard all of these questions and more from clients over the years as we've tried to help them deal with issues related to food cravings.

WHAT'S IN A CRAVING?

Simply stated, if you've ever had an intense desire to eat a particular food—anything from icy kosher dill pickles to salty potato chips coated with creamy onion dip to rich fudge almond ice cream—and you can't concentrate on your work, get to sleep, or even relax until you've eaten this, then you have experienced what is called a food craving. While there is no evidence that nutritional deficiencies cause these powerful urges, cravings may be the result of our reaction to stress.

"Wait a minute. I thought only pregnant women get food cravings." Pete complained of an uncontrollable yearning for hard-salami-and-cheese sandwiches late each night after starting his new job. The yearning quickly increased his weight by nine pounds, not to mention his LDLs (the "bad" cholesterol).

Sorry, Pete. The reality is that you don't have to be pregnant or even female to have special urges for certain foods. Cravings happen to most of us—male and female alike—whether we like it or not. While many people think food cravings are a detriment, they are normal and a part of life, especially of today's high-tech stressful life. Most of us, however, don't crave nutritional powerhouses like broccoli or spinach.

When we told Pete that his craving for salami-and-cheese sandwiches was probably related to the stress of his new job, he couldn't believe what we were saying. "You mean I'm eating to soothe my work anxieties, then gaining weight as a result?"

Perhaps subconsciously he was. In the midst of craving certain foods, whether during times of distress, like Pete, or not, we have many clients who come to us specifically for help in overcoming cravings. Most want to know why they crave these foods, if these desires present a nutritional problem, and how to control these cravings for optimal weight management.

RESTRICTION LEADS TO OVERINDULGENCE

We have found that cravers can be divided into three distinct categories, whether male or female, and we have provided you with a food craving assessment and quiz on pages 49–50 to help you identify your particular style. But it is important to know that even though you may fit into a specific category, everyone's craving style is different. What soothes the stress for one person may not work for someone else. For example, Barbara found that sugar soothed her workday anxieties, while Pete leaned toward fats (salami and cheese). Other cravers find that they desire salt to pacify their moods. During stressful times, Cathy leans toward french fries, and Susan prefers chocolate.

Not surprisingly, the problem with resisting a craving is that usually when you deny yourself something that you want so badly, you are likely to break down and eat more than you would have in the first place. People like Barbara who crave sugar and feel guilty eating it, often try to resist sweets completely, then end up eating too much.

The good news is that although sugar does not provide nutrition for your added calorie expense, it is not harmful. Sugar does not cause cancer, heart disease, osteoporosis, or diabetes. It does cause cavities, but other carbohydrates like bread or rice do, too. The concern with splurging frequently on high-sugar foods has to do more with what you are missing nutritionally by eating sweets than what you are getting in return. It's common knowledge that you won't find many antioxidants, phytochemicals, or fiber in your favorite cookie or ice cream (see Stress-Less Strategy #1 for why you need them), and that a steady diet of sugar cannot lead to optimal health and energy.

As a rule of thumb, eating any food occasionally is okay; it's the everyday choices that affect disease risk. Suppose you crave pizza, hot dogs, or hard salami, like Pete. These foods contain fat and particularly saturated fat; high fat intakes are related to diseases like cancer and heart disease. Some studies might frighten you away from eating certain foods, such as hot dogs or processed luncheon meats, for fear of getting cancer. While eating these foods on a daily basis might affect your risk of disease, for most healthy people, allowing yourself to have these "treats" once in a while will satisfy your craving without injuring your health. You may also try the low-fat versions of these foods. For some people, eating these is a good substitute. Others would rather have a little of the real thing.

So, while eating the craved food occasionally may not hurt you nutritionally, if you have other health concerns, you need to be aware of the total picture. Check with your doctor or nutritionist for individualized consultation.

THE EAT PLAN IS ABOUT ENJOYMENT

The EAT Plan is about stopping the guilty feelings associated with cravings and allowing indulgence. As you begin to implement the stress-less strategies, the first message we want you to hear about coping with cravings is that this urge for foods you love may be a signal that you are not getting enough fun out of what you regularly eat.

"I never knew that eating is supposed to be fun!" Caroline appeared stunned when we told her that what she had been doing habitually at least three times a day for thirty-three years was supposed to be enjoyable. "I always dread eating because I know I'm either going to gain weight from the extra calories or become ill from some unknown chemical or additive that causes cancer or heart disease."

Please turn off the news, and put your feelings of dread aside. We give you permission to lighten up when it comes to putting your fork to your mouth. The bottom line is that none of these foods you crave will cause you great nutritional harm, if you eat them occasionally. We believe that food is meant to be enjoyed, and in the last decade we seem to have left this enjoyment out of nutrition. Life's too short not to have some fun!

So what's the jury's verdict on cravings? There are a number of current theories, and it's important to examine each of them to see if they fit your unique style.

COMMON CRAVING THEORIES

THEORY #1:
CRAVINGS ARE CAUSED BY LIMITING FOOD

In other words, you want what you can't have. If we told you that in the EAT Plan you can never again eat ice cream, how long would it take before that was the only food you craved? What if we told you that the all-American hamburger was totally off limits with the EAT Plan? This, in itself, would make some of you immediately close this book.

The problem arises when we restrict a food because we think it's bad for us. Then we start to want that food, and a lot of it. Take potato chips as an example of a commonly craved food. You may refuse eating chips for weeks, knowing that 10 chips provides 140 calories and 8 grams of fat and, after all, who can eat just 10? Yet, in a weak moment, you eat potato chips and usually too many because you believe you may never get them again. After you eat too much, you feel guilty, so you go back to the restricting phase (see Figure 2.1). No more chips for you. While this restriction/indulgence pattern is unconscious, once you can identify your craving pattern, you can stop the progression.

Imagine a world where all food is okay, so you don't ever have to think, I can never eat that again. Now, again, we are not telling you that all foods are the same nutritionally, but we are saying that with the EAT Plan you can eat some of all foods without being a nutritional wreck.

THEORY #2: WE GAIN COMFORT FROM CRAVED FOODS

As children, we learned that certain foods are special or comforting. If you fell down and skinned your knee as a child, chances are that your mother or father said, "Let's have a cookie to make it feel better." Is it any surprise that when you have a stressful day as an adult, an entire bag of cookies might take away the sting?

We associate the cookies with comfort. You might also associate chunky chicken pot pie, steaming meat loaf and whipped potatoes, or creamy banana pudding as giving consolation on a stressed day. There are a lot of other so-called comfort foods, and they are different for each of us. Some of our favorite comfort foods are old-fashioned and make us think of home, like fried chicken, candied yams, or blueberry cobbler. When we crave these foods, are we really craving a little comfort in our fast-paced lives?

Figure 2.1

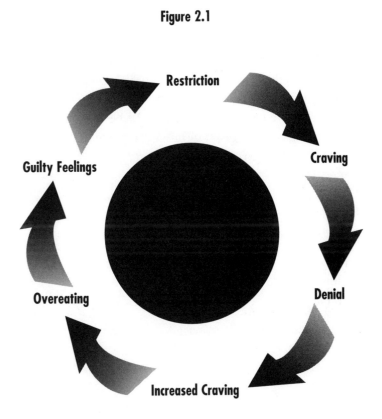

Ten Most Common Comfort Foods

Chicken and dumplings	Ice cream
Chicken pot pie	Macaroni and cheese
Chicken soup	Mashed potatoes with gravy or butter
Cookies	Meat loaf
Cupcakes	Pudding

THEORY #3: MISSING INGREDIENTS IN OUR DIET
CAUSE FOOD CRAVINGS

"I must be low on calcium because I crave ice cream," Teresa rationalized after consuming most of the half-gallon of ice cream. Fred reported that his diet must be low in protein, and that is why he constantly orders the double cheeseburger at McDonald's.

As Teresa and Fred claimed, are our bodies really trying to tell us something when we have food cravings? Maybe, and maybe not. The idea that cravings are the result of missing ingredients in our diet has not been verified by the research, yet it could be true in some cases.

One example of this theory is the idea that we crave chocolate because we are deficient in magnesium. Ginah told of eating a Snickers bar every night before bedtime because she heard that magnesium was important for a healthy heart and this was her "favorite way to get this mineral." While chocolate does contain the mineral magnesium, we have not seen any lower magnesium levels in people who crave chocolate versus people who do not. One must question if we craved chocolate for the magnesium, wouldn't we also crave black-eyed peas, oysters, or spinach? As you can imagine, we have not had one client report craving these foods.

THEORY #4: HORMONES AFFECT FOOD CRAVINGS

Becca craved rich Godiva chocolate each month: "Without fail, when PMS starts, so does my craving for Godiva." It's interesting that women report more food cravings around the time of their menstrual period or around the menopausal transition. A revealing study by Dr. A. M. Rossignol at Oregon State University reported that chocolate consumption and foods and beverages high in sugar particularly were associated with the time immediately prior to the menstrual period. This time is called the luteal phase of the menstrual cycle. It's also the time when some women report mood changes, usually for the worse, like sadness, shortened attention span, or just plan crabbiness. We know of clients who have eaten entire one-pound bags of M&M's or half a box of chocolate-chip cookies during this time. These cravings may be linked to the hormonal changes that fire the menstrual cycle. Estrogen levels fall in the luteal phase and progesterone levels increase. Both of these hormones have been linked to changes in brain chemistry affecting the neurotransmitter serotonin. Serotonin is associated with a calming, anxiety-reducing reaction. So during the luteal phase, serotonin levels are decreased and that is linked with the mood changes, depression, irritability and lethargy, and an increase in appetite, particularly for carbohydrate-rich foods such as chocolate, cakes, cookies, or ice cream.

Ten Most Commonly Craved Foods with PMS

Cake	Doughnuts
Candy	Ice cream
Chips	Nuts
Chocolate	Pastries
Cookies	Pies

THEORY #5:
SEX MAKES A DIFFERENCE IN FOOD CRAVINGS

In our survey of more than 1,000 adults, we found the most commonly craved foods for women were sweets, with chocolate ranked number one, and the most commonly craved foods for men were sweets, then salty or protein foods. One recent survey of women reported that 50 percent claimed they would rather have chocolate than sex. Now that's some craving! Women reported that their favorite forms of chocolate were candy, followed by ice cream, and fudge topping. Men's chocolate preferences were chocolate cream pie and chocolate cake. So there does appear to be some sort of difference due to sex.

Sex Differences in Food Cravings

Women	Men
Cake	Chips
Candy	Chocolate
Chips	Deli sandwiches
Chocolate	Nuts
Cookies	Pizza

THEORY #6:
SATISFYING CRAVINGS RELAXES OUR BODIES

Perhaps the most recent theory on food cravings has to do with the food-mood connection. This means that foods we crave affect our brain chemistry in such a way that we feel calmer and less anxious after eating. In our survey, women reported they were more likely to change their eating habits when they were anxious, sad, or bored, while men reported that they were more likely to change when bored or lonely.

Eating itself is (or should be) a calming, pleasant, social experience. Because we eat on the run so often in our fast-paced lives, the calming aspects of eating may be long gone. The research of Dr. Judith Wurtman of Massachusetts Institute of Technology (MIT) reports that selecting certain types of foods, such as carbohydrates rather than proteins, may actually calm us down, giving almost a self-medicating effect. Could this mean that the reason chocolate-chip cookies are so appealing is because of the change in brain chemistry they produce?

Chocolate particularly may produce a positive mood state. In her book *Why Women Need Chocolate*, nutritionist Debra Waterhouse reports that the sugar in chocolate boosts serotonin while the fat increases endorphins, another brain chemical associated with positive mood. This may explain why people report a feeling of happiness or contentment after eating chocolate.

THEORY #7:
FOOD CRAVINGS ARE CAUSED BY BRAIN CHEMICALS

Landmark studies at Rockefeller University by Dr. Sarah Leibowitz have shown that two specific brain chemicals affect our cravings. One is neuropeptide Y and the other is galanin. Leibowitz's studies point to a revealing truth: We eat what we are. This means that the different foods that we crave may be influenced by neurochemicals in the brain.

Neuropeptide Y has been directly linked in animal studies to the amount of carbohydrate we eat. Dr. Leibowitz reported that cortisol, a hormone produced during times of stress, has the ability to increase the desire for carbohydrate by increasing the production of neuropeptide Y.

Another neuropeptide, galanin, is associated with the intake of fat in Leibowitz's animal studies. The more galanin produced, the heavier the animal will become. In addition, galanin is affected by the hormone estrogen. Estrogen increases the production of galanin and makes us want to eat and deposit fat. So our increased calorie intake around the menstrual cycle and during puberty may be related to increased galanin production.

Leibowitz also reports that the level of these chemicals is different at different times of the day. Neuropeptide Y has its greatest effect on appetite early in the day, after our overnight fast. Neuropeptide Y is increased after any self-imposed period of deprivation such as dieting. So it is no wonder we found cereal, toast, or fruit, foods high in carbohydrates, to be the most common breakfast foods. Stress also increases the amount of neuropeptide Y. Again, it's not surprising that dieters and people under stress reach for carbohydrate foods, such as breads, sweets, pasta, and cereals. After lunch, the desire for fat increases as a way of storing calories in anticipation of the overnight fast to come. Galanin levels peak with our heaviest meal at night.

How does this relate to stress eating? Stress is associated with increases in neuropeptide Y but not galanin. The effect of stress on eating may not be the same throughout the day and seems to vary for different people, which is why some eat more and some eat less under stress. Someday, we may be able to tell in advance by looking at these brain chemicals who is at risk to overeat and who may eat less in response to stress.

THEORY #8: CRAVINGS ARE THE RESULT OF THE STRESS RESPONSE

Ah! Now we can get to the theory you've been waiting for—the one that explains why you would kill for a cookie, especially after a stressful day at the office or being stuck at home on a rainy day with energetic kids.

The stress response itself results in an increased desire for carbohydrates to give us the energy for the fight-or-flight response (see Chapter 1). Carbohydrate foods like breads, cereals, pastas, and fruits provide us with the fuel that the body needs to work. When under stress, we need energy to deal with the demands placed on the body. All carbohydrates provide a fairly rapid source of energy by raising blood-sugar levels. However, did you know that "stressed" is "desserts" spelled backwards?

REACT POSITIVELY TO CRAVINGS

No matter which of these theories appeals to you as a cause of cravings—and they may all play a role—you can gain a feeling of control over your cravings by learning to react positively when the desire hits. With the EAT Plan, you will learn that at times you can eliminate the craving altogether but at other times, you should just relax and give in. Yes, this means that you have permission to eat crispy fried chicken or Mom's just-baked oatmeal cookies once in a while. The EAT Plan gives you license to balance your life—to strike a balance between resistance and indulgence—so that cravings no longer pose a nutritional or weight-management problem.

Which foods would you "kill for"? Use the following list to

assess your favorite food cravings, and write how you feel after eating each food.

The following Craving Assessment and Craving Quiz will give you great insight into your particular type of craving.

CRAVING ASSESSMENT

List Your Craved Foods   **Your Feeling**

1._____   _____

2._____   _____

3._____   _____

4._____   _____

5._____   _____

6._____   _____

7._____   _____

8._____   _____

9._____   _____

10._____   _____

CRAVING QUIZ

1. I crave particular foods
   - ____ never
   - ____ rarely
   - ____ occasionally
   - ____ frequently
   - ____ daily

2. When I crave particular foods, they are mostly
   - ____ sweets
   - ____ salty foods
   - ____ protein foods
   - ____ other

3. I eat the foods I crave   _____ never

                                      _____ rarely

                                      _____ occasionally

                                      _____ frequently

                                      _____ daily

4. My cravings are the strongest during the

                                      _____ morning

                                      _____ midmorning

                                      _____ noon

                                      _____ midafternoon

                                      _____ evening

5. My cravings occur when I am

                                      _____ anxious

                                      _____ bored

                                      _____ worried

                                      _____ sad

                                      _____ angry

6. My cravings are strongest during specific times of the month.

                                      _____ Yes

                                      _____ No

7. My cravings are strongest when

                                      _____ I've eaten too much

                                      _____ I've eaten too little

                                      _____ I'm on a diet

                                      _____ I'm depriving myself

                                      _____ I feel fat

8. My cravings are for comfort foods.   _____ Yes

                                          _____ No

9. My cravings increase when I'm under stress.

                                      _____ Yes

                                      _____ No

This survey will enable you to identify your craving pattern. Now, depending on your responses, check the following to see under what Craving Category you fall.

CRAVING CATEGORIES

SUGAR CRAVER

Chances are if you are female, you crave sweets. In our survey, we found women to be more likely to crave sweets than men (52 percent of women versus 32 percent of men). Perhaps this is because of the latest theories relating carbohydrates, which include sweets, to stress. This gives credence to the Comfort Theory (Theory #2), as sweets can have a calming, anxiety-reducing effect. This may also be related to the Deprivation Theory (Theory #1), which says that we want what we can't have.

In our survey, 49 percent of all women questioned reported cutting out sweets to lose weight. The problem arises when you cut way back on sweets or eliminate them when reducing calories. The result is strong cravings for sweet foods.

The frequency of the craving is an important clue to your motivation. If you crave a food often but try never to eat it, then you may be in the deprivation/restriction mode (Theory #1). That could explain why your sugar cravings are so frequent.

With the EAT Plan, you will learn to have the food you crave once or twice a week in a reasonable portion, then watch the cravings diminish. Use the chart on page 49 to assess your favorite cravings for sweets. Then review the following examples of sweets that can be worked into your weekly nutrition plan without fear of weight gain or nutritional deficiency. Feel free to try these or your own favorites in similar quantities.

Craved Sweets	Serving Size	Calories	Fat Grams
Hershey's Kisses	3 pieces	75	4
Snickers Miniatures	1 piece	43	2

Craved Sweets	Serving Size	Calories	Fat Grams
Caramels	5 pieces	150	3
Butterscotch hard candy	5 pieces	112	1
Life Savers	5 pieces	45	0
3 Musketeers	1 bar	249	8
Milky Way	1 bar	251	9

SALT CRAVER

Even though you might picture men chomping away on pretzels and nuts while rooting for their favorite football team, you may be shocked to know that women also crave salty foods. This craving may occur around the time of the menstrual period because of estrogen's effect on the antidiuretic hormones, vasopressin and aldosterone, which can cause fluid retention. If you are a female, it's no news to you that women typically gain one to three pounds prior to their periods and that the weight is extra fluid. The shocking news is that some women gain as much as twelve to fifteen pounds. One client, Lois, had two sets of clothes, one a size ten and the other a size twelve for her preperiod time.

Craved Foods High in Sodium

Cheese	French fries
Chips (potato, corn)	Nuts
Cold cuts	Pickles
Crackers	Popcorn
Fast Food	Pretzels

PROTEIN CRAVER

If you crave protein foods, chances are you are a male carnivore. Through our survey, we have found that only 11 percent of women reported craving foods in this category while 32 percent of men longed for protein. A study at the University of Michigan School of

Public Health asked overweight men and women to list the foods that taunt them the most, and they listed both sweet and nonsweet foods. The common link was food high in fat. Men seem to crave fat from meaty food like pizza, cheese, or burgers, while women crave fat from cakes, candy, and other sweets.

Who do people crave foods high in protein? According to Dr. Judith Wurtman at Massachusetts Institute of Technology, protein foods have been associated with a feeling of increased alertness, concentration, and performance.

Fat Content of Craved Protein Foods

Food	Calories	Fat Content in Grams
McDonald's Big Mac	560	32
Cheddar cheese, 1 oz.	114	9
Bologna, 1 slice	73	7
Hot Dog	144	13
Pizza Hut Supreme, 2 slices	540	26

TO SNACK OR NOT TO SNACK?

No matter what your age or sex, most people indulge in their cravings for snacks. In 1990, the Snack Food Association reported that Americans consume 4.72 billion pounds of snack foods, at a cost of more than $12 billion. Other studies have found that most people interviewed told of snacking at least once a day, 97.8 percent of seniors reported eating between meals, and 99 percent of other groups reported eating between meals. Most people snacked in the afternoon, while seniors snacked more frequently in the evenings. Not surprisingly, 80 percent of the groups chose taste rather than nutrition as the basis for their choice of snack. Fruits, chips, popcorn, cookies, and candies were favorite afternoon snacks. Americans preferred salty/crunchy snacks, and eating snacks at home, while another survey indicated that the single favorite all-around snack item was ice cream. Stress-less Strategy #4 will help you make the most of your snack attacks.

WAKE-UP CALL

There is a growing body of evidence that cravings may be our bodies' way of getting our attention, causing us to think more carefully about what we're eating, when we're eating, and what situations cause us to eat. We designed the EAT Plan to put you in control. Remind yourself that to succeed with the EAT Plan, you will have to do some homework. As you learn what situations are making you "kill for a cookie," you can learn to deal with these powerful impulses and make the decision whether to eat one or not.

chapter   3

————•————

MY DIET IS A DINOSAUR

You'd have to agree that we live in a wonderful age, a time of medical discoveries and new technology. Yet, even though cutting-edge research on nutrition is constantly being revealed by the media, for most of us our eating habits border on prehistoric. This happens when you eat the same way for years and years, not necessarily because it is good for you, but because it is out of habit or the way you grew up.

Christopher came to see us because his boyhood eating habits were creating health problems for him at midlife. It seemed that as his position escalated up the corporate ladder, so did his stress levels and his weight. "My doctor says that my weight is too high," he said at the consultation. But upon looking at his lab results, his weight was not the only factor that was elevated. So were his blood pressure, choles-terol, and triglycerides—all important risk factors for cardiovascular disease, and Christopher had a history of this disease in his family.

Christopher did not exercise, except walking from his car to his office each day. "Breakfast? It's been the same since high school," he told us. "I grab two glazed doughnuts and a thermos of coffee [thirty-six ounces] at a convenience store down the street."

And Christopher's dinosaur dieting habits didn't stop there. "I drink another two cups of coffee when I get to the office. Then because I'm trying to reduce my weight, I try to skip lunch or just grab a package of cheese crackers, along with a diet cola. I do eat a balanced dinner every night."

Balanced? The menu he described included buttery potatoes, fried pork chops, vegetables cooked in bacon fat, and hearty biscuits, topped with what he called a "light" dessert—ice cream. After consuming his only meal of the day around 7:00 P.M., Christopher would begin his nightly exercise routine: channel surfing while dozing in his new leather recliner.

Over a period of two decades, Christopher had gotten in the dinosaur-diet habit of eating foods high in fat, along with no physical activity. Why? Because it was what he had always done. But we convinced Christopher that these habits can be broken and new ones learned.

The results of a variety of studies prove that to succeed with weight loss, we must make the dinosaur dieting habit extinct and make positive lifestyle changes. This includes revamping our eating habits, activity level, and attitude.

If you are like many of our clients, perhaps you do not feel confident unless you are dieting or skipping meals as Christopher did in an attempt to lose weight. Linda said she feels "fat and out of control" unless she is rigidly depriving herself of food. "The only time I feel in control of my eating and my life is when I'm on a strict diet, even though it leaves me feeling cranky, hungry, and deprived."

Linda's enslavement to "diet deprivation" is shared by many. At any one time, 50 million or more Americans think that they need to lose weight and are trying to lose weight with diets that just don't work. But while starving to lose weight or depriving yourself of your favorite foods may produce a few pounds of weight loss, this is usually very short-term. Starvation or food deprivation never results in long-term weight management because diet deprivation almost always leads to bingeing on what you forced yourself to give up initially.

Our survey of more than 1,000 men and women found that when Americans are trying to lose weight, 69 percent cut out fat, 61 percent reduce portions, 49 percent eliminate sweets, 14 percent skip meals entirely, and 6 percent cut carbohydrates. While it appears that most people know the healthful way to lose weight is by cutting fat and controlling portions, why is it that America's weight problem is on the rise? Could it be that we cut fat without controlling portions? Or do we understand how to lose weight but we don't have time to do it? Perhaps we are just too stressed out to care.

DIET: A FOUR-LETTER WORD

What does the word *diet* mean to you? The real definition is "nourishment" or "nutrition," implying health and vitality, but somehow most highly promoted diets are anything but nutritious, and they certainly aren't healthy. In fact, highly promoted diets such as the high-protein and low-carbohydrate diet or low-calorie liquid diets can be downright dangerous if followed for a long period of time.

Here is what our many clients have shared with us about their diet experiences:

A diet means

- if it tastes good, it must be bad for me
- deprivation
- starvation
- denial
- cravings
- depression
- elimination
- hunger pangs
- a lifetime sentence
- a four-letter word

Yes, for most of us, *diet* truly is a four-letter word. Why? Because the typical diet does not represent a realistic lifestyle change. No matter what the supermarket tabloids guarantee, two weeks of deprivation dieting cannot make up for years of out-of-control eating, poor nutrition, and lack of exercise. As one of Susan's students said, "The word *diet* typically describes the way I feel. Drop the 't,' and I feel like I'm going to die."

Published surveys show that the success rate of most diets attempted by obese people is barely 5 percent; so 95 percent of diets don't work to keep the weight off. Why the relapse after dieting? Some claim that the newly discovered fat gene is to blame; others point their finger at the set-point theory. Set-point weight is the weight that the body tends to visit and revisit. It seems that the set point can only be changed by altering the metabolism.

Now go ahead and dust off your walking shoes because this alteration will not occur through diet but by a consistent, ongoing active life, which includes exercise and activity. Traditional dieting alone breaks down your muscle mass, which is the metabolically active tissue. Exercise alone may not be the key either. If you eat more calories than you burn, you will not shed the pounds. Researchers feel that the winning strategy is the combination of a healthy nutrition program and a fitness program full of exercise and activity.

It is interesting that when we tell overweight clients who have a lengthy history of dieting that we're going to teach them a new way to lose weight, that is, eat and lose weight, they become quite uptight. Dieting, even though it resulted in denial of the very foods they loved without permanent weight loss, had become an integral part of their daily lifestyle.

For Lauren, a thirty-nine-year-old mother and trial attorney, dieting was a way of life. She described being on her first diet at the young age of six. "My pediatrician instructed my mother to put me on a diet because I was a chubby child," Lauren said. "All I remember about my childhood and teenage years is Mom serving me salads, skim milk, and melba toast for dinner. She never knew that I would sneak back into the kitchen later to grab a handful of cookies."

The reality is that there is no quick fix for years of failed dieting.

The good news is that losing weight and controlling your weight are not even about diet and deprivation. You're probably reading this with your mouth open, wondering if this is really true. It is. For decades, we've been taught the wrong way to lose weight. In the past five years, comprehensive scientific studies have shed light on the impact of deprivation diets on weight loss, and the findings have consistently held true: *Diets don't work!*

Starting today, we want you to eliminate the word *diet* from your vocabulary totally and focus instead on nutrition with our EAT Plan— and this means, first and foremost, eating, and eating all day long.

Figure 3.1

DINOSAUR DIET

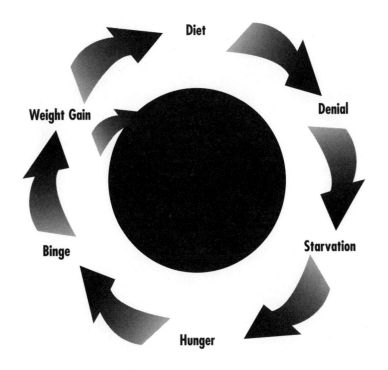

BARBIE: AN UNREALISTIC ROLE MODEL

You may be thinking, Okay, if diets really don't work, why does everyone I know still diet? It must provide some benefit; after all, diets are big business.

Dieting *is* a big business, so big that $50 billion a year is spent on

Figure 3.2

THE EAT PLAN

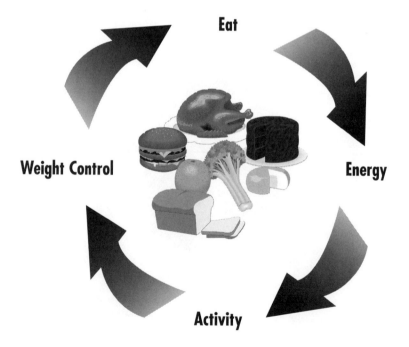

diet products and diet programs. Compare this with the $34 million spent each year on obesity research. Talk about misplaced priorities.

While both men and women diet, studies show that twice as many women diet as men. Interestingly enough, we have found that most men typically diet for health reasons, such as losing weight to lower their cholesterol or reduce high blood pressure, while women diet for appearance. After all, it is no news to you that Barbie was and still is the first role model that many young girls are drawn to. However, for most women to look like Barbie they would have to be six feet tall, decrease their waist size by six to seven inches, push those excess inches up to their chests, and pose in the "high heel" position all the time. This sounds unrealistic and uncomfortable to us.

Not only do men and women diet for different reasons, they also gain weight in different places. Women tend to gain in the hips and thighs, while men gain weight in the middle. The problem is that the apple shape is more at medical risk than the pear shape. Pear-shaped women: Don't relax yet, for you may turn into apples at the onset of menopause. Because of changes in hormones (lower estrogen levels), many pear-shaped women will start to gain this android fat, or fat in the middle.

If you don't know where your "fat point" is, then grab your measuring tape and calculate your waist/hip ratio. It is simple to do. Measure your waist (in inches); then divide this by your hip measurement (in inches over the widest part).

Recommended Waist/Hip Ratio

Women	Men
.8 or less	.95 or less

You are not the only one interested in this measurement. Obesity researchers are using waist/hip ratios to look at risks of developing different diseases. For example, for women with waist/hip ratios greater than .8, there is a greater risk of breast cancer, heart disease, high blood pressure, and diabetes. For men, waist/hip ratios greater than .95 are associated with increased risk of heart disease, high blood pressure, and diabetes.

How's Your Nutrition?

"Quit stalling! I've grabbed my waistline, now tell me how to make it shrink," Patrice demanded as she sought guidance in losing the weight she'd gained with her third child. Before we tell you what *does* work for long-term weight loss, we need to look at your nutrition history and tell you why people gain weight.

When was the last time you had a nutrition checkup, if ever? As registered dietitians, it amazes us how people would never forget to take their dogs or cats to the veterinarian for shots or never drive for years without an oil change in their cars. But these same people rarely take the time to think about themselves and the way they treat their bodies.

Use the Nutrition Checkup that follows to reassess your eating and lifestyle habits. A "yes" answer to any one of these questions is reason enough to take an up-close and personal look at yourself and your overall nutrition and food intake, not just at weight gain or weight loss.

NUTRITION CHECKUP

Answer yes or no to the following to see how your eating and lifestyle habits measure up.

Yes   No

____ ____   1. You constantly feel the effects of stress, such as headaches, backaches, stomach distress, or tension in the neck.

____ ____   2. You are not pleased with your current eating habits.

____ ____   3. You feel chronically fatigued or routinely lack the energy to be at your best.

Yes   No

_____ _____ 4. You eat on the run and survive on what we call hit-or-miss meals or grab-it-and-go meals. This means that you don't think about your body, nutrition, or the calories involved.

_____ _____ 5. You have a slow metabolism and seem to maintain your weight on very little food.

_____ _____ 6. You struggle with creeping waistlines and dislike your body image.

_____ _____ 7. You routinely go on and off diets, only to regain the weight you lost.

_____ _____ 8. You exercise rigorously, compulsively, and/or excessively.

_____ _____ 9. You obsess about food and have undesired binges that seem out of control.

_____ _____ 10. You have high cholesterol, diabetes, or high blood pressure or have relatives with these conditions.

LIVING WITH EXCESS BAGGAGE

The reality is that as we age, our metabolism slows down. Unfortunately, so does the activity level of most people. The problem begins when the amount of food we eat does not decrease. In fact, for most of us, the amount of food we eat usually stays the same or increases, resulting in unwanted pounds or excess baggage to carry around.

Obviously, then, the really big issue for almost all of us is the reality that the golf cart and automobile get more use (or exercise) than we do. In fact, many studies show that it is not unusual for Americans (adults and children) to watch three to five hours of television per day instead of engaging in exercise or physical activity.

Obesity is a rapidly increasing concern in America today. We can attest to this truth with an ever-growing client list of people who want to know how to lose weight. According to statistics released in 1995 from the third National Health and Nutrition Examination Survey (NHANES III), which provides data gathered from 1988 to 1991, one-third of Americans are overweight. This is equal to 58 million people in our country carrying around the stress of excess pounds. The really shocking statistic is that between the NHANES II survey of 1976–1980 and the NHANES III survey of 1988–1991, the percentage of people ages 20 and older considered to be overweight jumped from 25.4 percent to 33.4 percent. And all of this weight gain took place in a society inundated with fat-free foods and miracle diets. Could it be that our "fat phobia" has made us lose sight of realistic eating habits? Perhaps we have forgotten that fat-free is certainly not calorie-free.

Although studies revealed that we ate less fat as a percentage of total calories (34 percent as compared to 40 percent in the mid-1960s), the data from NHANES III also revealed that we consumed 100 to 300 more calories per day. It doesn't take a degree in nutrition to calculate that eating more calories over time without expending extra energy will result in weight gain.

WHAT IS YOUR SET-POINT WEIGHT?

Our clients tell of struggling for months with all types of deprivation diets, yet once they lose a few pounds their bodies seem to gain it back immediately and return to their original weight. Some clients feel that no matter what they do, their weight seems to stay or be most comfortable at a certain figure (and not necessarily the hourglass look they are seeking).

If you are wondering if your brain is preprogrammed to tell your thighs to awaken automatically whenever you eat a cookie or ice cream, then you don't want to dismiss this theory in the weight gain/weight loss arena. The set-point theory has been around for at least twenty years and is seeing a flurry of research to bring it back to the forefront. A fascinating study conducted by Rockefeller University and reported in the *New England Journal of Medicine* kept track of obese and nonobese people and found that the obese people had a tough time maintaining weight loss. Simply stated, their own metabolism may work against them.

The set point may be regulated by the adipostat in the brain, which increases your appetite when you lose a few pounds in order to put them back on. Could this theory also be tied to the discovery of the fat gene? The gene, called the ob (for obesity), produces an ob protein called leptin, derived from the Greek root *leptos*, meaning "thin," that circulates in the blood. Leptin decreases appetite by causing you to feel full and may also increase energy output. Obese people may have a problem with the receptor for leptin, so their appetites do not respond.

THE PROBLEM WITH WEIGHT CYCLING

Time and time again, we have seen clients whose appetites haven't changed since young adulthood, but their bodies and metabolism have, and they gain more and more weight as time goes by. Perhaps this is one main reason highly advertised diets are so popular, especially those that "guarantee" to make you look and feel ten years younger and weigh ten pounds less in just two weeks so that you can wear that new outfit, be seen at your class reunion or whatever event may be motivating you to lose the unwanted weight. The problem occurs when you continually lose and gain the same weight over and over again.

For those who have lost and regained the same twenty-five pounds for a decade, this weight cycling could be heading you for disaster. Research has suggested that a repeated weight loss/weight gain with dieting increases body fat. It is suggested that the up-and-down of weight loss and gain replaces muscle with fat. When weight is regained, it is gained as fat, which in turn lowers the metabolic rate. Thus, every time you start over, you start from a harder place. You have a higher percentage of body fat and a more sluggish metabolism. This is by no means a reason to give up the weight-loss effort, but it is a strong point in the favor of lifestyle changes over time versus diets that promise quick loss.

You Can't Turn Back the Clock

Not long ago, one of our clients came for a weight-loss evaluation after gaining thirty-nine pounds during her pregnancy. Even though she had lost most of the weight, she was still about eleven pounds over her previous weight. "I want to look the way I did in this photograph." Shelly, who wore a size eleven, handed us a picture that appeared to have been taken at her high school senior prom fourteen years before, when she wore a size five evening gown.

When we responded that no matter how much she dieted, she probably would never look exactly that way again, she was astounded, saying, "But that was the only time I felt good about myself."

While body-image issues are more of a woman's concern than a man's, one recent British study found that women who work out regularly gave themselves a higher rating in terms of health and attractiveness than those women who did not exercise very often. Interestingly enough, the women exercising weighed ten to twelve pounds more than the nonexercising group. These findings make sense because we know that two of the great rewards of regular exercise are a toned look and increased feelings of self-esteem (see Chapter 5 for more on the benefits of exercise).

Some of us might blame our weight on family history. Look at the size and weight of your parents and grandparents. If that is a scary thought, we want you to know upfront that you do not have to succumb to becoming overweight. It is true that as we age, the body's metabolism rate (the rate at which our bodies burn calories) slows down. But that does not guarantee that growing older means growing fatter.

No matter what your age or weight history, we believe that it is time for an attitude adjustment for the millions of men and women who have suffered through decades of diets, denial, and deprivation with resulting weight gain. But before we describe to you the key to long-term weight management, as outlined in our EAT Plan, let's understand the real truth behind losing weight.

TRUTH OR CONTROVERSY?

Today, there is more information available than ever before on weight loss. In spite of the latest knowledge, there is still controversy among researchers as to exactly how we gain and lose weight and what we should eat. Intriguing controversy arose when some researchers claimed that the majority of overweight people are insulin resistant and that carbohydrates cause them to overproduce insulin, which results in an increased appetite, and thus leads to an increase in body fat.

As such, too much insulin could play a significant role in increasing the risk for certain diseases such as heart disease, hypertension (high blood pressure), or diabetes. But the prevailing question is, Does too much insulin actually make you fat? In one landmark study conducted by Dr. G. M. Reaven at Stanford University, results indicated that a high-carbohydrate, low-fat diet does produce higher insulin levels than a low-carbohydrate, high-fat diet. But as long as the calories remain the same on either diet, there does not seem to be a change in weight.

Others agree and claim that insulin is not the culprit that makes you fat, but actually it is being overweight that can cause you to become insulin resistant. When you lose those excess pounds, the problem with insulin resistance seems to be resolved. Even people who are diagnosed with diabetes as adults seem to have more stable blood glucose levels when excess weight is lost. Diagnosing diabetes is a much simpler job than determining if someone is insulin resistant. Again, Dr. Reaven suggests that a high triglyceride level (above 200) and a low HDL level (below 35) may be indicators of insulin resistance. High blood pressure and excess body weight may also tie into this set of symptoms referred to as Syndrome X.

Then there are new studies that claim the medications you take to treat illnesses such as depression, high blood pressure, or allergy (all can be triggered by stress) can contribute to weight gain—even if you are eating low-fat, low-calorie foods and exercising. According to the *Physicians' Desk Reference* (PDR), a widely used compilation of drug information, more than 100 prescription drugs may cause weight gain in some people. Apparently the drugs can cause a change in the body's metabolism, allowing fewer calories to be burned and more to be stored as fat.

So what's the bottom line? (No pun intended.) The truth in losing weight is that total calories as well as total fat are important. And the long-standing truth is that calories over and above what your body uses in a day, regardless of where they come from, will make you gain weight.

HOW TO MAKE THE DINOSAUR DIET EXTINCT

Now that you understand why you may have gained weight from stress eating and why you need to quit dieting in order to lose this excess weight, you can begin to learn more about the EAT Plan. We ardently believe that life is too pressured and harried to follow a rigorous diet, depleting you of energy or enjoyment. We want you to forget about being skinny or at an unrealistic weight, find peace with your body image, and drop the guilt trip society feeds you for not being its definition of perfect. The EAT Plan is about letting go and enjoying life once again.

CHANGE YOUR ATTITUDE ABOUT DIETS

As we rethink our attitudes about dieting, let's also take a look at throwing out the garbage known as "good food" versus "bad food." Remember when you had that piece of Kentucky Derby pie that your Aunt Rosie always makes on your birthday? You probably heard that annoying bird on your shoulder start to chirp, "I can't believe you sat there and ate that entire piece of pie and then licked the knife. Those calories will just go directly to your stomach, and you'll have a new inch to pinch by morning."

With our EAT Plan, you can finally stuff a sock in that nagging bird's mouth and eat one of the foods you dream about as you rid yourself of the guilt regarding good food versus bad food. After all, we know that avoidance breeds obsession. Don't believe us? If you give up one of your favorite foods because you are trying to go on a diet, what is the first thing you notice? For most of us, we want that food now more than ever. We think about it continuously; we dream about it; our mouths salivate as we visualize it in our mind. Finally, because it has become such an obsession, we *have* to have it—and a lot of it, to the point that we binge or overeat.

The problem arises when we become judgmental about food, when we lose the experience of enjoyment and the taste of a variety of foods. Our judgment about good food versus bad food can even be carried over into our self-esteem. Haven't you punished yourself heartlessly for eating that one piece of fudge? Perhaps the media feeds this frenzy with the constant reporting of research as good or bad in terms of how it affects your health. Sure, that sensational method works as a hook and draws you in, but we believe that life is too precious and short to become neurotic when it comes to food choices.

FOR WOMEN ONLY

Each day we are subjected to Madison Avenue's idea of the "perfect" body. As if that were not enough, even well-meaning friends and family members add their own suggestions about how we must look to be "our best." But these images of perfection have done a great disservice to men and women today, and we must forget this Barbie image. Most of us will never look like that perfect teen model because of genetics anyway. And—let's not forget to mention for those who are over forty—you are not only fighting genetics, you must confront the added reality of gravity and aging. Comparing yourself to the Barbie image at any stage of life is self-defeating and does nothing for your morale.

"Oh, I don't care if I look like Barbie," Lynnette, a forty-three-year-old mother of three teens, commented while grabbing her leg. "But this cellulite on my thighs is disgusting! How do you lose weight just in your hips and thighs?" You start by learning what that cellulite is composed of. Cellulite is just another word for fat or lipid or adipose tissue; all are one and the same, and spot reducing, such as repeated leg lifts, does not work. Weight loss happens over the entire body.

Under a microscope, cellulite looks just like any other fat cell, but on your thigh it takes on the appearance of cottage cheese because it is trapped fat stored beneath the skin. It particularly takes on this appearance as we age and the skin loses its elasticity, letting the fat show through. Because of this unsightly look, we are willing to try bee pollen, vinegar, blue-green algae, grapefruit only, pasta only, all-protein diets, and a host of other scams that don't work—just to lose weight. The sad truth is that many people would rather be dead than fat.

We know that it is easy to set yourself up for defeat by falling prey to the model-thin look of the fashion magazines. But we also know that if you focus on your own body and what is a realistic, healthy weight for you—one that you can live with—you can look great, feel terrific, and have a vitality for life.

BODY IMAGE ASSESSMENT

Yes   **No**

_____ _____   1. I think my body is ugly most of the time.

_____ _____   2. I avoid looking at mirrors because I don't like what I see.

_____ _____   3. I find it difficult to enjoy outdoor activities such as swimming because I'm embarrassed about my physical appearance.

_____ _____   4. When I go shopping, I'm always self-conscious when trying on clothes or telling the salesclerk what size I need.

_____ _____   5. I feel guilty about my weight and shape most of the time.

Yes	No	
____	____	6. Not a day goes by that I don't think about my body and its appearance.
____	____	7. When people look at me, I know they are also thinking that I have an ugly body.
____	____	8. When I go through fashion magazines, I am envious of the models.
____	____	9. I know that if I had a more attractive body, I would be happier and more successful.
____	____	10. Every time I go anywhere, I compare myself to other women to find someone with an uglier body.

IGNORE THE MYTHS

If you answered yes to any of these questions, your self-esteem could use a boost. Our clients who use the stress-less strategies in our EAT Plan report not only changes in nutrition and activity, but feel better about themselves, as well.

Despite the research on healthful nutrition and how it affects weight loss, confusion still prevails. The following statements seen in the headlines are enough to make you shake your head in frustration:

- Fat is bad for you but olive oil is good.
- Saturated fat is bad, but chocolate is not as bad as you think.
- Eat fat-free foods, but some carbohydrates might make you fat.
- Calories don't count as long as you are eating low-fat foods.

Now don't let all of these seeming contradictions make you feel as though you want to toss in the towel. Remember that nutrition is a young science and all of this commotion is a sign of the intense research in an area of great promise for your health and weight management. Probably beta-carotene-boasting carrots could be considered a bad food if that is all you consumed for a day. No doubt the time is right for a paradigm shift from good food/bad food to eating, enjoyment, and energy.

THE NEWS ON WEIGHT-LOSS AIDS

"Can't you give me a little pill that will help me lose weight?" Britt begged us to recommend a diet supplement after reading about some "miracle" fat-burning pills in a popular women's magazine.

Before you get too excited and reach out your hand, here's what we told Britt—the honest truth: You can't get something for nothing, and some weight-loss aids are not safe. Now you might look at the sales of diet aids (more than $3 billion worth a year are sold) that claim to help burn fat, and laugh, saying, "Come on! They sure must work for somebody."

In addition to being expensive, diet aids can make all kinds of health claims that have never been proven by scientific studies. Unfortunately, the effects on the body can be just as unsafe as prescription drugs used inappropriately. For example, ephedrine and mahuang are common ingredients in diet supplements. Ephedrine is a decongestant found in some OTC (over-the-counter) cold, allergy, and asthma remedies and acts as a stimulant in the body. It can raise heart rate and increase blood pressure by constricting blood vessels, which is a concern for people with high blood pressure (hypertension), heart or kidney disease, and diabetes. While you may hear claims that ephedrine increases thermogenesis (the rise in metabolic rate after you exercise or eat), it is the stimulant effect that makes you "feel" as though it is burning fat. Mahuang is a Chinese herb that contains ephedrine so the same concerns apply as with ephedrine.

We like to explain it this way: If you go shopping for a new car, one of the factors that may influence your decision is the window sticker touting the miles per gallon of gas on the highway and around town. If you buy a car promising thirty-six miles per gallon on the highway, drive it on a few trips, and determine the mileage to be six-teen miles per gallon, how are you going to feel? Probably taken for a big ride, so to speak, and not very happy with the car dealership or manufacturer for misleading you.

As a savvy consumer, you may want to look twice at products that tout their ability to melt away your excess fat. Although the future may be quite promising for the use of certain herbs, right now you will get a huge helping of testimonial promises without much sci-entific evidence to back it up. What can be really scary is that the people selling these weight-loss aids may have absolutely zero nutri-tion or medical training yet they are selling you products that at best don't work for long-term weight control and at worst may be harmful to your health. Do you want to be the guinea pig in their experiment?

In the EAT Plan, we will give you some exciting "weight-loss aids" that you may not have considered before, starting with activity, exercise, and creative changes in your lifestyle. We know that you can get rid of unwanted weight caused by stress eating.

THE FUTURE OF WEIGHT LOSS

Some scientists are trying to develop drugs to combat compulsive eating and weight. With all the research and scientific data, it has become apparent that both compulsive overeating and bulimia have been linked to low serotonin levels. Several studies suggest that treating bulimia with antidepressant drugs to increase serotonin levels may decrease the number of binge episodes. The thought is that depression associated with bulimia is eased as the serotonin level increases. Serotonin also regulates appetite and thus reduces the desire to eat uncontrollably.

For society as a whole, the greater interest is in developing drugs to work for obesity and compulsive eating. The challenge is to find a drug that is safe for long-term use because to be effective for weight control, these medicines would have to be taken for a long time. The drug dexfenfluramine, which is said to increase brain serotonin levels, could help overeaters cut back on food. The antidepressant drug

Prozac is currently being studied, as it has had the unanticipated side effect of short-term weight loss. It is in the group of drugs that increases the brain's serotonin level. Could these drugs or others like them decrease your appetite and produce positive feelings of well-being along with weight loss? There are other drugs on the horizon to help you lose weight by reducing dietary fat absorption, reducing carbohydrate absorption, increasing metabolic rate, or reducing food cravings. How well these will work, only time will tell.

So if you've been wondering if your brain overrules your body when it comes to your weight, the answer could most definitely be yes. Perhaps it is our stressed-out, fast-food, grab-it-and-go society that is more the demon behind the belly bulge than anything else. But the situation is not one of doom and gloom. Rather, our EAT Plan will enable you to change your priorities and give yourself permission to *eat*—once and for all.

chapter 4

———— ◦ ————

CALM ME DOWN AND
PUMP ME UP

Isn't it rewarding that researchers have finally acknowledged what many parents (and nutritionists) have been telling us for generations, that is, "You are what you eat." Some have even called this new era of research psychonutrition, while skeptics are calling it "too early to tell." In our practices, we have promoted psychonutrition for years, counseling clients and teaching seminars on how to beat stress eating as you eat to feel great and maximize performance.

If someone were to tell you, "You are what you eat," what would you be? A deli sub smothered in Italian dressing? A New York cheesecake? Smoked pork barbecue? When we shared this information with Ashley, a seminar attendee, she commented, "If we are what we eat, then I guess I'm just one sweet, homemade chocolate-chip cookie."

While we don't mean this literally, the connection between what we eat and what happens in the brain to influence mood, behavior, or performance is one of the hottest areas of research today. Simply put, our daily choices of food make us better able to deal with stress. As you will see, that is an important focus of our EAT Plan as you learn to control stress eating. Likewise, when we are overly stressed, it is usually our harried mood that dictates our food cravings.

After taking the Craving Quiz on pages 49–50, you may look at the food-mood equation and now agree that how you feel throughout the day influences your food choices and cravings. However, this chapter will bring you to a new realization about how to cope with stress in your life. Although what Popeye believed when he touted spinach as creating an instantaneous improvement in behavior and physical ability is not true, the connection between food and perfor-

Figure 4.1

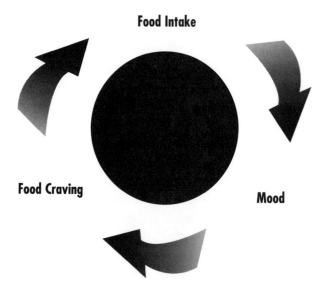

Food Intake

Food Craving

Mood

mance is being more clearly defined. Remember how this childhood hero became stronger, tougher, and better able to deal with Bluto after gulping a can of spinach?

Don't worry. We aren't going to hold spinach as the stress-eating cure-all (although it is high in cancer-fighting phytochemicals), but in the EAT Plan we will follow the same premise that you believed as a child, except that Popeye will now represent you, spinach will represent food, and Bluto will be the stress that you face each day.

FEED YOURSELF TO COPE WITH STRESS

In the past decade, the idea that certain foods alter your mood by influencing the level of brain chemicals called neurotransmitters has received a lot of attention from researchers. Many other factors from heredity to drugs or alcohol can influence the level of these brain chemicals. In addition, it was discovered that three neurotransmitters—dopamine, norepinephrine, and serotonin—are produced in the brain from components of the foods we eat every day. Neurotransmitters are the chemicals we use to get messages from cell to cell. Think of a neurotransmitter as a cellular phone. Our diet dials this "neurotransmitter phone," and it can increase or decrease the amount of these chemicals resulting in mood or performance changes.

> Norepinephrine and Dopamine = Alertness Brain Chemicals
> Serotonin = Calming Brain Chemical

Research by Dr. Judith Wurtman at MIT has revealed that people are more alert when their brains are producing the neurotransmitters dopamine and norepinephrine. These brain chemicals are significant as is the neurotransmitter serotonin, which is associated with a calming effect and reduced anxiety, and can lead to drowsiness.

Based on scientific studies, we know that serotonin is also the neurotransmitter most closely linked to dietary influences. A stable serotonin level in the brain is associated with a positive mood state or feeling good over a period of time.

When looking at the effects of serotonin, it also appears that women may have a greater sensitivity to changes in this brain chemical. Mood swings during the menstrual cycle, menopause, or following the birth of a child are thought to be caused by the action of the changing hormones on brain chemicals.

The key foods that increase production of serotonin in your brain are carbohydrate-rich foods (see Figure 4.2). Many kinds of carbohydrate-containing foods can produce a serotonin response, from candy to popcorn to pasta. That explains why we may feel

Figure 4.2

HOW YOUR BRAIN PRODUCES THE CALMING CHEMICAL, SEROTONIN

Eat carbohydrate food

Increase blood sugar

Increase the amino acid tryptophan relative to other amino acids

Entrance to your brain

Increase brain tryptophan

Increase brain serotonin

drowsy after a big pasta meal for lunch, since a rise in serotonin in the brain is associated with a drowsiness effect.

THE ROLE OF PROTEIN

As we mentioned previously, there are two other important brain chemicals that appear to be influenced by the foods we choose: dopamine and norepinephrine. Unlike serotonin, these chemicals produce a feeling of alertness, increased ability to concentrate, and faster reaction time. Think of the alertness chemicals as turning on a light-bulb, making you feel brighter and more focused.

Although there is still some debate as to how this mechanism works, the two prominent theories are:

1. Serotonin production is blocked by the consumption of protein-rich foods, resulting in increased alertness.
2. Dopamine and norepinephrine may be produced through the dietary consumption of protein.

For your brain to increase production of dopamine and norepinephrine, protein-rich foods are the key (see Figure 4.3).

Through the research of Dr. Wurtman and others, the idea of manipulating mood and performance through food choices was born. We have shared this research with clients with excellent results. Although each person's response is different, everyone finds that food affects how they feel, and how they feel affects their performance. You, too, can find your response to particular foods and then use that information to curb stress eating by following Stress-Less Strategy #2, becoming an Active Mood Manager.

Figure 4.3

How Your Brain Produces the Alertness Chemicals Dopamine and Norepinephrine

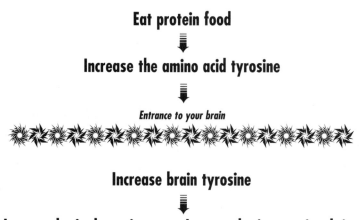

Eat protein food

Increase the amino acid tyrosine

Entrance to your brain

Increase brain tyrosine

Increase brain dopamine ⟶ Increase brain norepinephrine

SOME GROUNDS FOR CONCERN

Many factors influence how alert and energetic we are each day, and when we talk about using food to give a boost of energy and to be more alert, we mean it in a positive way. But there is another food substance that most of us use on a daily basis to affect our mood and performance that we don't think about in that way. You guessed it—caffeine.

Caffeine is a central-nervous-system stimulant used by more than 80 million Americans. In small doses, this food substance can improve your mood and make you more mentally alert. The problem occurs when people overuse caffeine or have a sensitivity to its effects, for it can lead to anxiety, insomnia, or restlessness. This substance is just what you don't need if you are trying to calm down and de-stress your life! And, if you stop using caffeine cold turkey, there are some nasty withdrawal symptoms, the most common being severe headaches.

Previously researchers thought that only those people who consumed large amounts of caffeine would suffer withdrawal. But some of the latest studies have found that as little as one cup of coffee every morning, if missed, can produce withdrawal symptoms, ranging from the initial headache to irritability, depression, fatigue, nausea, and flu-like symptoms. The onset of these symptoms is usually twelve to twenty-four hours after the last dose of caffeine, and withdrawal can last up to five to seven days.

Caffeine is the only food ingredient we know of that actually mimics the stress response. With caffeine, you get an initial increase in heart rate, blood pressure, and glucose availability to the brain, which affects alertness. For most people, one or two cups of coffee, or just 100 to 200 milligrams of caffeine, can improve performance, reduce fatigue, and act as a stimulant following the slump many people experience after eating a large meal. But let's get back to the reason why you are reading about the EAT Plan: If you're already stressed, do you really need another boost to experience the stress response? Probably not.

With our busy schedules, we have found that decaffeinating is a productive way to decrease stress effects. To avoid the effects of withdrawal, you need to reduce caffeine to a minimum (less than 100 milligrams a day), which is less than 5 ounces of coffee per day. This reduction of caffeine used to be much harder until the advent of the many decaffeinated teas, soft drinks, and coffee products now on the market.

As you focus on the adage "You are what you eat," it's important to assess honestly the amount of caffeine you get every day, and adjust this to a minimum or, if you prefer, none at all—to keep caffeine from adding to your stress in harried times.

Caffeine Content of Favorite Products

Foods	Serving Size	Caffeine in Milligrams
Milk chocolate	1 oz.	1–15
Bittersweet chocolate	1 oz.	5–35
Chocolate cake	1 slice	20–30
Beverages		
Coffee, drip	5 oz.	110–150
Coffee, perk	5 oz.	60–125
Coffee, instant	5 oz.	40–105
Coffee, decaf	5 oz.	2–5
Tea, 5 min. steep	5 oz.	40–100
Tea, 3 min. steep	5 oz.	20–50
Hot cocoa	5 oz.	2–10
Cola soft drink	12 oz.	45
Drugs		
Anacin, Empirin, Midol	2 tabs	64
Excedrin	2 tabs	130
No-Doz	2 tabs	200
Dexatrim	1 tab	200

GET YOUR RHYTHMS IN SYNC

Because our EAT Plan is a lifestyle approach to making stress work for you, understanding how food affects your moods is just one part of the puzzle. We have found that it is also important to understand your body clock and distinguish whether you are a night owl or an early bird. As you will find out in Stress-Less Strategy #2, depending on your internal body rhythm, you can learn how to eat to calm down or eat to energize.

After reading over the checklist on page 86, Caroline identified herself as an early bird, waking up at five o'clock each morning to go for her morning walk, getting to work by 7:00 A.M., then working all day at her job as a magazine editor. Of course, she was fast asleep by nine o'clock each night, when many people are just sitting down to dinner. "I have no brain when it comes to late-afternoon or evening meetings," she told us. "If I could talk to writers at sunrise, there would be no problem. However, when I have to negotiate payment for articles late in the day, I find it hard to be sharp and focused."

With a little assistance from some high-protein foods at lunchtime and midafternoon, Caroline was able to work with her body clock instead of against it. On days when she knew she'd have a late conference call with a writer or an editorial meeting, she would eat a high-protein lunch, such as chicken breast and vegetables, followed by a late-afternoon snack of low-fat cheese. She found that she did, in fact, have a brain; she just needed to give her neurotransmitters a jolt of protein to become more alert and energetic.

Like Caroline, all of us experience fluctuations in our body temperature, heart rate, sleep stages, and hormone secretion, all without realizing it, every day. These fluctuations translate into a pattern of either early rising and morning alertness or staying up late and feeling most alert at night. These synchronized changes in internal body characteristics are called our circadian rhythms. Circadian rhythm can be described as a separate, individually synchronized internal rhythm that affects how we function each day. It determines our daily sleep cycles, performance and alertness, moods, and even our gastrointestinal functions. If you think this is a matter of choice or training, think again. Many people have tried to shift their rhythm to match their partner's, but to no avail.

Our usual internal cycle runs for a period of twenty-five hours. However, since there are only twenty-four hours in a day, as we are too often reminded, we have to adjust. We adjust by using external cues such as light or darkness, temperature changes, humidity and barometric pressure, and, perhaps, even eating patterns. These cues allow us to reset our circadian clock every day and adjust to changes that might throw us off, such as jet lag, sleeping late, staying up late, or working a night shift. These adjustments are not always easy, so symptoms can occur that indicate that we are out of sync, such as stomach upset, fatigue, weakness, irritability, insomnia, or a shortened attention span.

Circadian rhythm is also affected by age. Researchers at Duke University studied memory in college students and older adults aged sixty-six to seventy-eight. Regardless of age, many subjects reported no difference between morning and evening ability. Of those who did have a preference, young adults preferred evening, while the older adults were all morning people. However, when memory tests were given, there was a difference in scores based on time of day. With morning testing, both groups scored the same, but later in the day, test scores were 40 percent lower in older subjects and 50 percent higher in younger students.

Sleep is one of the most important factors affected by our circadian rhythm, and if you are having trouble sleeping at night, you have company: Most adults over age forty express the same problem, a problem that increasingly worsens with age and higher levels of stress. As you adopt the EAT Plan into your lifestyle, it is important to understand that sleep changes are a common symptom of stress, whether you wake during the night or are unable to fall asleep because your mind is racing with everything you need to do.

One revealing study found that Americans have cut their sleep time by 20 percent in the last century. This reduction of sleep time is a problem for the majority of adults, who need at least seven hours of sleep each night. One study found that those adults who slept only six hours each night experienced more frequent health problems, and over a period of nine years, these shorter sleepers had a 70 percent higher mortality rate.

There is one thing that is certain about sleep: The impulse to sleep is overwhelming, and we spend almost a third of our lives doing it. Before you can become an Active Mood Manager in our EAT Plan, it is important to understand the five different stages of sleep.

Stages of Sleep

Stage 1: Light sleep

Stage 2: Moderate sleep

Stages 3 and 4: Deep sleep

Stage 5: REM sleep (rapid eye movement) or dream stage

Recent studies have shown that Stages 3 and 4 appear to be the most important ones for physical recovery. If sleep disturbances occur during these stages, you will wake up feeling tired and may complain of muscular aches and pains. REM sleep is associated with psychological well-being and feeling refreshed upon awakening. People who are deprived of REM sleep complain of irritability and moodiness.

In addition to its effect on mood, sleep deprivation can have another very important effect similar to the effects of stress: It weakens the body's immune function. Dr. Michael Irwin studied healthy male volunteers and found that one night of sleep deprivation (a 45 percent reduction in total sleep time) resulted in a nearly 30 percent reduction in cellular immunity. Sleep, therefore, is being looked upon as a basic defense mechanism to preserve health.

How much sleep do you get? Do you wake up frequently at night? Or are you really a night owl forced to perform in an early bird society?

DISCOVER YOUR BODY RHYTHM

Most of us know that we are either an early bird or a night owl. But if you are unsure, use the following checklists to determine your circadian style.

EARLY BIRD TRAITS

_____   1. I wake up before the alarm goes off, ready to tackle the day.

_____   2. I feel more energetic and productive during the morning hours.

_____   3. Often I'm up before daylight working on projects.

_____   4. I am least energetic and alert during evening hours.

_____   5. A typical bedtime would be around 9:00 to 10:00 P.M.

NIGHT OWL TRAITS

_____   1. I only wake up when the alarm is blasting.

_____   2. My ideal workday would begin at noon.

_____   3. It takes several cups of coffee for me to function in the morning.

_____   4. I am most productive and alert at night.

_____   5. A typical bedtime would be after the late night news.

NO ONE CAN DO IT FOR YOU

We want you to realize fully that no one but *you* can deal with your stress. However, we are going to teach you to become your own Active Mood Manager as you learn to make foods work *for* you instead of *against* you. For many of us, learning to eat to feel more energetic and alert, less tired, less apprehensive, and better able to deal with stress, along with working with our own circadian rhythm, will require a new way of thinking, a change in lifestyle. But we know that when you feel in control of your life and your emotions, you will be less likely to stress-eat, and that is the goal of the EAT Plan.

chapter 5

HELP! I'M TIRED AND I CAN'T GET MOVING

"Sure, I could combat stress," Julie said honestly, "if only I had some time and energy. I read the magazines and know I should exercise. But after working full time and coming home to two teenagers, I'm so stressed out that walking around the block is the last thing on my mind."

Sound familiar? Aren't we all like Julie in that we know we should get up and get moving, yet something holds us back? Without incorporating a regular exercise and activity program in your lifestyle, stress eating is tougher to conquer.

"Oh, I run every day," Bill, a seminar attendee, smiled mischievously as he said that the only running he did was far away from his company's fitness center. Rest assured, Bill, wherever you are, you are not the only middle-aged person who runs from physical activity. According to the Centers for Disease Control and Prevention (CDC), 56 percent of men and 44 percent of women between ages 18 and 29 exercise regularly. But these numbers drop to 44 percent and 40 percent, respectively, among people 30 to 44. The likelihood of obesity also increases during the thirty-something years: Only 16 percent of women and 20 percent of men ages 18 to 29 are obese, compared with 25 percent and 32 percent, respectively, of 30-to-44-year-olds.

In our survey of more than 1,000 men and women, we found that 33 percent seldom exercise and 18 percent do so only twice a week. Twenty-five percent exercise three times a week, while only 11 percent exercise five times a week and 7 percent every day. Time is a reality check for all of us. There just never seems to be enough of it, and exercise is the first item to go, yet it is one of the most beneficial things we can do for our body and mind. It makes sense that if we feel good, life looks better and is easier to deal with.

WHY WE DON'T EXERCISE

We've heard the gambit of reasons from stressed clients as to why they avoid exercise, including:

"How can I exercise? Have you looked at my daily calendar? With two preschoolers, along with working, I have to schedule time to go to the bathroom."

"Sure, I'd exercise if you'd get me some energy pills."

"Sorry, just thinking about exercising makes me depressed."

"Oh, I did try once. I joined a gym last year and walked the track on the first day. I was so out of breath that I thought I would die, so I quit."

"There's no way this tired body can exercise. It takes all my energy to feed my children after teaching school all day."

"If you would take over my business and get rid of my stress, then maybe I'd feel like exercising."

Perhaps the most pointed statement was made by Phyllis, the vice president of a prestigious bank, who said, "I need a commitment. If you will guarantee me that exercise will help me lose weight and reduce my stress, I'll be first in line."

We admit that we've said some of the same things over and over again, but the jury is in on exercise as one of the best personal changes we can make to combat weight gain, fatigue, anxiety, depression, and stress eating. Even though most clients tell us that they just do not have the energy to go and "work it out," once they begin the regular program of activity and movement we teach, the increase in energy and the decrease in stress eating speak for themselves.

"Why does walking for thirty minutes reduce stress eating?" you might ask. Because exercise increases the body's brain chemical that enhances our positive mood. Not only does physical activity increase alpha waves, which are associated with relaxation and meditation, but exercise also acts as a displacement defense mechanism for those who are literally "stressed out." If you have ever participated in a lengthy period of aerobics or walked for several miles, perhaps you know the benefit of this displacement defense mechanism. Isn't it difficult to worry about daily stresses when you are working so hard physically? Your mind is focused on the activity, not the problems you face each day. It makes sense that if you feel more in control of your life after exercise, ten out-of-control bingeing is less likely to occur.

TAKE A WALK AND CALL ME IN THE MORNING

"It still does not make sense," Ken said, "how exercise can make me feel more relaxed on a stressful day. I am so keyed up after a day at the office that the only things that relax me are a couple of beers, my recliner, and the sports channel." We explained to Ken what stress was doing to his health and how exercise was his prescription for unwinding.

After hearing our explanation, Ken was still skeptical, so we'll share with you what finally convinced him. Have you ever accidentally dropped a can of cola? What happens when you quickly pull the tab to open it after it has been shaken from the fall? Of course an explosion occurs, and a sticky one at that. Now, take this same can of cola, only carefully open the tab so that just the smallest amount of fizz escapes. When you open a pressurized can this way, the force is greatly reduced as the excess is released.

We want you to consider daily stress as the "fizz" or carbonation that activates when the can of cola is dropped; your body is like the

Figure 5.1

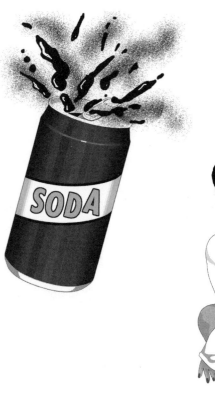
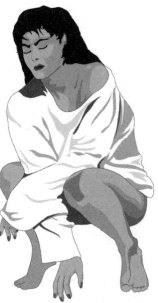

can of cola. In this regard, stress has to happen only for a minute or two before you will react with the fight-or-flight response, as discussed in Chapter 1. If stress is ongoing, day after day, and you have not released the accumulated adrenaline that is making your heart pump, then just like the cola, you will explode. This "explosion" could result in a physical response, such as ongoing fatigue, panic attacks, hypertension, ulcers, or weight gain or loss due to stress eating or not eating.

There is a solution for this buildup of adrenaline, and it has to do with letting some "fizz" escape each day before it has a chance to burst. The solution is exercise and activity. This is the only mechanism other than the passage of time that will allow stress hormones to escape so they do not build up and literally explode in your body, causing all sorts of internal problems.

WELLNESS WORK SHEET*
DO YOU NEED TO IMPROVE YOUR LEVEL
OF PHYSICAL ACTIVITY?

Medical Clearance

In general, if you are under thirty-five, have no physical complaints, and have had a medical checkup within the past two years, it is probably safe for you to begin an exercise program at your current level of physical activity and gradually increase it. To determine whether you need to consult your physician, read through the following list of statements and check any that are true for you.

____ I am not feeling well.

____ I have a specific health concern.

____ I am over 20 percent above my desirable weight and much of the excess is body fat.

____ I have been sedentary for a long time.

*Material originally appeared in *Your Guide to Getting Fit*, 2nd edition, by Ivan Kusinitz and Morton Fine, published by Mayfield. Copyright © 1991. Reprinted by permission.

_____ I have a history of some type of cardiovascular disease.

_____ I cannot walk more than two miles.

_____ I have one or more of the following symptoms after exertion:

     _____ Chest pain

     _____ Dizziness or faintness

     _____ Gastrointestinal upset

     _____ Difficulty breathing

     _____ Shortness of breath for more than ten minutes after exertion

     _____ Lingering fatigue and difficulty in sleeping

_____ I am thirty-five or older and have a history of coronary heart disease risk factors:

     _____ Diabetes

     _____ Hypertension

     _____ High blood cholesterol levels

     _____ Cigarette smoking

     _____ A blood relative who had a heart attack before age sixty

If you checked one or more of these statements, you should consult your physician before beginning any type of exercise program.

Calculate Your Activity Index
1. Frequency: How often do you exercise?

If you exercise:	Your frequency score is:
Less than 1 time a week	0
1 time a week	1
2 times a week	2
3 times a week	3
4 times a week	4
5 or more times a week	5

2. Duration: How long do you exercise?

If each session continues for:	Your duration score is:
Less than 5 minutes	0
5 to 14 minutes	1
15 to 29 minutes	2
20 to 44 minutes	3
45 to 59 minutes	4
60 minutes or more	5

3. Intensity: How hard do you exercise?

If exercise results in:	Your intensity score is:
No change in pulse from resting level	0
Little change in pulse from resting level (slow walking, bowling, yoga)	1
Slight increase in pulse and breathing (table tennis, active golf with no golf cart)	2
Moderate increase in pulse and breathing (leisurely bicycling, easy continuous swimming, rapid walking)	3
Intermittent heavy breathing and sweating (tennis singles, basketball, squash)	4
Sustained heavy breathing and sweating (jogging, cross-country skiing, rope skipping)	5

To calculate your activity index, multiply your three scores:
Frequency ___ × Duration ___ × Intensity ___ = Activity index___

To access your activity index, refer to the following table:

If your activity index is:	Your estimated level of activity is:
Less than 15	Sedentary
15–24	Low active
25–40	Moderately active
41–60	Active
Over 60	High active

If your activity level is in one of the lower categories, review the components of your score (frequency, duration, intensity) to see how you can raise your score. Add to your current exercise program or devise a new one.

JUST A LITTLE BIT CAN HELP

Have we captured your attention? Perhaps you are agreeing at this point that while exercise is necessary to get rid of your stress, the "no pain, no gain" theory offers a good excuse to bow out totally. A recent issue of the *Journal of the American Medical Association* gave new recommendations from a panel of exercise experts assembled by the American College of Sports Medicine (ACSM) and the Centers for Disease Control and Prevention. The group of experts concluded that the no pain, no gain workout thought by many to be the only way to get really fit is *out*.

We've talked with numerous clients who didn't participate in physical activity because they thought that they had to exercise vigorously and continuously to reap benefits. According to this report, regular, moderate-intensity physical activity will provide substantial health benefits. Now how's that for a warm-up to exercise?

This regular, moderate-intensity physical activity is also the best prescription for regular weight management or weight loss. The Centers for Disease Control, along with the American College of Sports Medicine, made recommendations on the types and amounts of physical activity needed for health promotion and disease prevention, and these groups concluded that every adult in the United States should strive to accumulate 30 minutes or more of moderate-intensity physical activity every day of the week. This 30 minutes can accrue during the course of the day to burn approximately 200 calories, which is equal to a brisk 2-mile walk. Even if you don't change what you eat, if you burn 200 extra calories each day this year, you can expect to lose 20 pounds.

You might choose to "accumulate" your activity time each day, and get your total exercise in short bouts such as walking short distances instead of driving, taking the stairs instead of the elevator, riding a stationary cycle while you watch the news, gardening, housework, yard work, dancing, or playing actively with your children. Yes, even mopping your kitchen floor counts as exercise. One of our clients, Diana, loved that suggestion. As a mother of four young children, keeping a clean house while working full time was probably her biggest stressor. Now she realizes that she gets the benefit of a clean house, reduced stress, and a tighter waistline—all with one activity.

Oh, did we forget to mention that women burn about 45 calories for every 10 minutes of passionate sex while men burn 60 calories? We'll leave that for you to ponder.

Common Ways to Burn 200 Calories a Day*

Activity	Minutes to Burn 200 Calories
Aerobics (high/low impact)	20
Bicycling (12 mph)	22
Cleaning	54
Cooking	72
Dancing (slow)	68
Dusting	82
Food shopping	60
Jogging (5 mph)	26
Making beds	82

*Based on a normal metabolic rate of a healthy 130-pound woman.

Activity	Minutes to Burn 200 Calories
Mowing lawn (power)	58
Stationary cycling (10 mph)	32
Tennis (doubles)	52
Typing	178
Vacuuming	34
Walking (3 mph)	54
Walking (4 mph)	36
Watching television	154
Weight training	40
Weeding garden	38

THINK LEAN AND STRONG

Meredith had followed our EAT Plan for six weeks, but she wanted more. She needed to drop the fifteen pounds she'd gained during a recent job transfer. We asked Meredith to add strength training to build lean muscle mass, the metabolically active tissue that helps to speed up your metabolism, even at rest. While it is true that the metabolic rate slows down with age, the fact that we are less active doesn't help. Strength training is a great answer, and we're not talking about bench-pressing 200 pounds. As you will learn in Stress-Less Strategy #3, we want you to start with five- to fifteen-pound weights, then develop a realistic strength-training program where you can lift ten to fifteen repetitions, doing two to three sets a time. This type of strength-training program can result in greater lean body mass in contrast to the average American adult, who loses about six pounds of lean body mass each decade of life after age thirty. Strength training is an addition to, not a replacement for, aerobic exercise.

You may be thinking, How can I find the time for even more activity? Maybe you are already doing more than you think. Cathy carries boxes, books, and a heavy briefcase through airports each week and has greatly increased her muscle strength while doing her regular work. Lifting groceries and heavy objects at home can also help if done regularly. Susan has implemented a strength-training program with free weights. She notices improved strength on the tennis court as well as ease in lifting heavy items, such as a twenty-pound bag of cat food for her hungry animals.

In addition to preventing sports injuries, strength training can be an aid in the prevention and reversal of osteoporosis (the loss of bone mass associated with aging) in older women. As a result, it can function in the prevention of falls and frailty. It seems that women over the age of fifty have much to gain from strength training by increasing bone mass and muscle strength. This is particularly important when you consider that one-third of all women who live to age ninety will break a hip and one-quarter of all woman over age sixty will suffer crushed vertebrae. If you want a more youthful profile, more muscle tissue, better balance, and better bones, consider strength training.

In one study where the women participated in two 45-minute strength-training sessions per week for 1 year, the women gained 3 to 4 pounds of muscle, lost 2 pounds of fat, improved muscle strength by 50 to 75 percent, and had a 1 percent increase in bone density, while the sedentary control group lost muscle and gained fat. Not only that, but balance improved by 14 percent in the exercise group while the control group had a decline of 8 percent in balance.

One of the most terrific findings was that the exercising women became more active over the year, becoming involved in leisure activities such as dancing, gardening, and walking—all great ways to keep a positive mood and alter the negative effects of life's stressors.

LIFE IS SO GOOD

Now that you are starting to get a glimpse of how activity diminishes the fight-or-flight response that goes hand-in-hand with stress and also helps with weight loss, there is still more good news. The latest studies confirm that we don't have to run to realize the exciting stress-reducing benefit of a "runner's high." When you engage in aerobic exercise such as bicycling, tennis, dancing, or even walking, not only do you alleviate stress and tension, but your body also produces and releases endorphins, marvelous "happy hormones" that are the body's natural opiates.

Endorphins work as the brain's natural painkiller, sometimes exerting analgesic effects more powerful than narcotic drugs. When you exercise aerobically, endorphins are produced that give you a sense of calm and well-being after the activity. The endorphins act as a fax machine between the brain and the body to influence mood and behavior. As the endorphin level increases, your outlook on life becomes better. People who exercise regularly claim that "the world looks so much brighter" after a workout. One client, who walked every night after work for an hour, told of her husband accusing her of having an affair with another man because she had such a pleasant grin on her face when returning. On the other hand, some clients say the grin is the result of being finished with the exercise.

Another terrific benefit, according to Dr. Adam Drewnowski of the University of Michigan, is that exercise—even as little as a brisk ten-minute walk—can curb food cravings.

> Endorphins = Positive mood

EXERCISE REDUCES DEPRESSION

Remember, as we discussed in Chapter 1, fatigue is a typical response to distress. When you are tired from stress, the last thing you want to do is be physically active, yet this is the time when you need to be. But fatigue can also be caused by depression or even serious diseases. If you are continually tired, it is important to rule out depression or illness as the source and see your physician.

Studies have shown that while depression affects 7 percent of the adult population in the United States, or about 15 million Americans, it appears that 13 to 20 percent of the general population has depressive symptoms. Some estimations are that as many as 25 percent of the United States population experience anxiety, mild depression, and other emotional disorders.

Depression is the most common psychiatric disorder in women and may affect as many as 20 to 26 percent of women and 8 to 12 percent of men. Although race and socioeconomic factors have not been clearly tied in, the incidence of depression is known to be highest in lower socioeconomic groups.

Several studies have tied severe depression to an increased risk of fatal heart disease. A recent study from the Centers for Disease Control and Prevention looked at 2,800 people from ages 45 to 77. None of the volunteers had heart disease when they entered the study, but about 25 percent said they had mild symptoms of depression. After 12 years, the depressed people had a significantly higher rate of heart disease and death. The people who felt the greatest sense of hopelessness at the beginning of the study had almost double the rate of heart disease and death as the nondepressed people.

Statistics indicate that only one-third of people dealing with depression seek assistance even though depression is treatable, particularly with the advances in medications that increase the brain's serotonin level and improve mood. But the good news is that exercise can help alleviate depression. In one revealing study performed on seventy-four depressed men and women at the University of Wisconsin in Madison, psychologist Marjorie Klein compared the effects of two forty-five minute running sessions a week with both meditation and group therapy. After twelve weeks, Dr. Klein found that exercise was just as effective in alleviating depression and that all three approaches reduced anxiety and tension.

EXERCISE PROMOTES WELLNESS

Especially for those of us who are constantly bombarded with daily stress, activity may be the key to protecting our bodies from disease. Scientific evidence links regular physical activity to a variety of mental and physical benefits. One study done at Harvard Medical School found that 80 percent of the students who were healthy engaged in regular aerobic exercise, while only 20 percent of the students who became ill exercised regularly. Another recent report in the *Journal of the American Medical Association* found that physically active adults develop and maintain a higher level of physical fitness than their counterparts who are sedentary. Research has shown the protective effects of physical activity in decreasing risk for high blood pressure, heart disease, diabetes, osteoporosis, anxiety, depression, and colon cancer. On the other hand, low levels of physical activity are tied to increased mortality rates. It has been estimated that 250,000 deaths per year in the United States, or 12 percent, are attributable to lack of regular physical activity. Daily activity improves heart disease risk factors and other health-related risk factors such as blood lipids (cholesterol, HDL, LDL), glucose tolerance, bone density, body composition, immune function, and psychological function.

The report also says that men are more likely to engage in regular activity, sports, and exercise than women. As we age, we also spend less of our time being physically active. People with higher levels of education participate in more leisure-time physical activities than do people with less education. What is the number one reason people do not participate in physical activities? No time. Look at Stress-Less Strategy #4 for creative ways to plan so that you can make time for *you* a priority each day.

"I haven't had a cold in years." When Rhonda told us that we were impressed. Can you imagine staying well year after year even during the grueling cold and flu season? Well, there's more to this immune power than just good genes. Regular exercise appears to have the benefit of stimulating the immune system and reducing the number of cold and flu episodes. One explanation seems to be in the increased activity of lymphocytes, called "killer cells," as a result of consistent exercise, as well as an increase in the amount of immunoglobulin found in the blood. Increases from 50 to 300 percent have been reported. Watch your workouts, though. Studies also show that when workouts become stressful or excessive, the body produces increased amounts of cortisol, which can inhibit the ability of certain immune cells to work properly.

William Evans of Pennsylvania State University suggests that older people have a blunted immune response to exercise, meaning that the body takes longer to recover from exercise and perhaps to adapt to all kinds of stress. He recommends that older people take 200 to 400 international units (IU) of vitamin E a day, for it seems to enhance the immune response. (See Stress-Less Strategy #1 for more information on the power of antioxidants.)

EXERCISE HELPS TO INDUCE RESTFUL SLEEP

One client, a retirement-age gentleman, came to us because he could not sleep and thought that learning to de-stress would help. This man had tried some over-the-counter sleep aids and was still not sleeping.

"Exercise was the only thing that helped me relax and sleep," Joe said. "When I worked full time, I was exhausted at night. But now that I'm home, I need that afternoon bike ride to sleep soundly at night." Joe now rides three miles a day and sleeps well at night.

Studies show that physical inactivity may contribute to insomnia by inhibiting our normal and rhythmic increases and decreases of body temperature. Regular exercise in the late afternoon or early evening eliminates this problem because it makes your body temperature rise and then fall (as you cool down). This aids in sleep because decreasing body temperature facilitates the onset of sleep and promotes deep sleep.

GET PHYSICAL AND LIVE LONGER

Exercise can also increase our life span. Researchers at the Cooper Institute for Aerobics Research in Dallas gauged fitness in about 13,000 men and women and divided them into five equal groups, ranging from the least to the most fit. Then the researchers followed them for an average of eight years. As the level of fitness

increased, fewer deaths occurred. Even being slightly more fit produced a significant drop in the death rate.

ALLERGIC TO SWEAT?

"There's no way I can exercise because I'm allergic to sweat."
Sally, a young woman who reminded us of Scarlett O'Hara, said. At
first we thought maybe something was wrong with Sally physically;
after all, sweating is a normal bodily function. However, when we
questioned her further, she laughed then said in the sweetest southern
drawl, "Oh, no, dears. My body can sweat, but I choose not to."

Sally's problem was solved quickly by sending her to a local
sporting goods store to purchase an electronic treadmill. Then, in the
privacy of her lovely air-conditioned home while watching her
favorite soap opera and with two fans blowing on her body, Sally
began walking two miles a day—and finally lost the twenty-four
pounds she had gained with a recent pregnancy.

Home exercise equipment is big business for those of us who
prefer to cocoon at night and on weekends. In fact, over $2 billion
worth of home exercise equipment is purchased each year, falling
into one of two categories: (1) equipment that strengthens the cardiovascular system; (2) equipment that builds muscular strength.

If you prefer to exercise out-of-doors, save your money. But for
those like Sally who refuse to sweat or who feel unsafe going out at
night to exercise, machines are the perfect solution. Especially when
the weather is bad or you keep late hours, the perfect piece of equipment can help you stay on track with your fitness program while
watching your favorite TV show.

ACTIVITY SHOULD BE PLEASURABLE

Most people think that going on a diet means exercising. As
people go off diets, they stop exercising, and a negative attitude

toward exercise begins. Exercise or physical activity then becomes a brutal form of punishment instead of a pleasure.

Reluctance to exercise becomes more of an issue when trying to lose weight is a person's entire reason for the activity. Physical activity should bring joy and be fun with a focus on pleasurable activities. Choose activities that can be part of daily life, such as walking the dog, gardening, making love, walking the mall, or taking a walk and gathering flowers along the way.

We know how easy it is to become disenchanted with yourself if you exercise for the sole reason of getting an ideal look instead of providing increased energy and positive self-esteem. But we also know that attitude is half the battle. As you change your attitude toward exercise and how it can change your life, it is important to understand that stress is 10 percent what happens to you and 90 percent how you react to it.

USE MIND/BODY TECHNIQUES

Not only can exercise be used to increase endorphins so that you feel better about life, but researchers in the field of psychoneuro-immunology (PNI) are revealing fascinating reports that "we are what we think." There are mind/body exercises we can do in the privacy of our home or office to feel calm and at ease, and the benefits of these techniques extend throughout the entire day, helping to curb stress eating.

Psychoneuroimmunology is a comparably new field and centers on the connection between the brain, the body, and the immune system. Health professionals in this field figure that between 90 and 95 percent of all health problems can to some degree be traced to the influence of emotions. Some are going so far as to say that an optimistic outlook, such as a feeling of control, may in some way protect against disease or illness and act as a valuable complement to conventional medical care.

In harmony with that belief, we all know that when we have peaceful thoughts, we tend to have a comparable emotional reaction and similar physiological reaction as well; we are in control of our life and our eating. When we have angry or anxious thoughts, we tend to be emotionally aroused, and consequently our physiological reactions are more dramatic, thus we are prone to bingeing on food. An increasing number of physicians, psychiatrists, and psychologists are acknowledging that the way we think, feel, act, and react can be a powerful determinant of physical and mental health.

As you will learn in Stress-Less Strategy #3, incorporating the following mind/body techniques in your daily life is not difficult. But before we teach you how to do this, it is important to know why they will help make stress work for you in the EAT Plan.

MUSIC THERAPY

Twenty-two-year-old Jen tells of de-stressing to the soothing harmony of the Indigo Girls. Rob, age thirty-nine, prefers the melodic New Age music of Danny Wright, while his wife, Sarah, prefers Tony Bennett. No matter what your age, music therapy has been proven to be an effective nonpharmacologic approach to reducing fear, anxiety, stress, or grief. It is just beginning to make its mark in stress management, yet many are already reporting music therapy as a great way to lower stress.

The effect of this natural tranquilizer on the human spirit can be tied to Pythagoras, the sixth-century-B.C. philosopher and mathematician who is thought to have been the founder of music therapy. In the 1940s, the Veterans Administration hospitals had volunteers who played their music for the wounded soldiers. The results were so positive that the VA added music therapy programs. Today, there are more than 5,000 registered music therapists in our nation who use music to soothe, and some speculate heal, physiological and psychological problems.

Music may have therapeutic value in working with patients coping with autism, chronic pain, head injuries, poor motor control, and learning difficulties to facilitate a change in behavior. Even surgeons reported performing better when they could select the music played in the operating room. Composer and researcher Steven

Halpern says that certain musical forms can transport the listener's brain into the alpha wave, a state of relaxation much like meditation.

A recent survey of 308 men and women found that exercising and listening to music were the most successful ways for them to get out from under a dark cloud. *The Journal of Personality and Social Psychology* reported that twenty-six psychotherapists rated music and physical activity as smart ways to enhance mood. Next time you need a mood mender, try walking for as little as ten minutes while listening to your favorite musicians.

Matching creative juices with technical lab studies, researchers and composers are turning out compositions, from classical music to babbling brooks, specifically designed to relax you and reduce mental fatigue and lower stress.

AROMATHERAPY

Aromatherapy is one of our favorite ways to relax after a stressful day of conducting seminars or meeting with clients. Susan prefers the fruity scent of raspberry, while Cathy finds the cooling fragrance of eucalyptus to be soothing. This type of "nose/body therapy" is an ancient art that uses highly concentrated oils, usually distilled from herbs, flowers, fruits, roots, grasses, leaves, and seeds, to affect our sense of smell and thus our sense of well-being. It is said that certain fragrances spark immediate reactions in our bodies and can possibly be beneficial in helping us to relax from days filled with stress, anxiety, and feelings of burnout.

Research is being conducted on aromas or scents and how they may alter one's mood and thoughts. Studies have been done on odors such as spiced apples, and this particular scent produced feelings of relaxation. These same studies show that other scents, such as lemon, make people more alert. Perhaps we should consider using lemon fragrance in the boardroom when major decisions are being made. What about spraying a spiced apple scent after the board meeting when stress hormones are raging? It just might work.

Research by Dr. Alan Hirsch at Rush-Presbyterian–St. Luke's Hospital in Chicago suggested that scents in food affect the urge to eat. When overweight people who were dieting inhaled a smell like Fritos corn chips, they lost an average of 4.17 pounds in two weeks. Those who inhaled no scent lost 1.59 pounds during that time. Dr. Hirsch reported that the smell of Fritos seems to fool the brain into thinking you are full even when no Fritos are eaten.

Lavender was used to perfume the baths of the Romans and for over 1,000 years in folk remedies. Interestingly enough, a recent report in *The Lancet*, a well-respected medical journal, indicated that lavender oil was associated with reduced symptoms of insomnia in the elderly and therefore could reduce the need for hypnotic drugs. Some of these drugs have significant side effects and have been prescribed for long periods of time. Although the number of people in the study was small, geriatric residents in a nursing home who had been prescribed tranquilizers for a couple of years had their sleep measured for six weeks. The medication was used the first two weeks, discontinued the next two, and the ward was perfumed with a diffuser and lavender oil the last two weeks. It seemed that although removing the medication reduced the number of hours spent sleeping, the scent of lavender produced the same amount of sleeping time as that obtained through medication.

Apples to calm down? Lavender to enhance restful sleep? Is aromatherapy an old wives' tale or does this work? Exactly how the scent-mood link works still remains a mystery. Researchers do know that when aromatic molecules waft into the nose, they hook onto receptors there and build electrical impulses that move up the olfactory nerves to the brain. These researchers feel that the optimum target is the limbic system, where memory and emotions are processed. At this time, there is widespread agreement that certain aromas help to increase the quality of sensory input for people, thus helping to reduce stress and the stress response.

GUIDED IMAGERY TECHNIQUES

For years, Elizabeth has been overreacting every time she feels pressure or deals with new situations, from taking a test in college to going out on a blind date to meeting with her new employer about a raise.

"For days before I have to face a stressful situation, I just imagine myself falling apart," she said. "Then I really do fall apart when it becomes a reality. My hands shake, my heart races; I want to run away."

Elizabeth can't spend her life hiding from social pressures, so our goal was to get her to relearn how to react. We told her, "The brain has no idea that a test is necessarily bad, or that a meeting with the boss is frightening. Your brain only knows what you tell it, and if you tell it something horrible might happen, it will react accordingly, triggering the fight-or-flight response."

Elizabeth learned to send positive signals to her brain with guided imagery. Also called visualization, guided imagery is considered a method of communication between body and mind that utilizes perception, position, and movement. It involves mentally seeing pictures of relaxing situations, such as a sunset on the beach, or a flowing mountain waterfall, especially during stressful times. Visualization also involves seeing yourself being successful, such as that meeting with your boss ending with a substantial raise in salary. Visualization uses the following thought processes:

- Vision
- Smell
- Taste
- Touch
- Position
- Movement

One researcher suggests that experiencing an event through imagination is equivalent to actually having the experience. Hmm . . . perhaps imagery could reduce a great deal of financial stress as you imagine being on that seven-day Caribbean cruise while in the comfort of your own home.

Elizabeth learned to trigger the power of her imagination as she used sights, sounds, feelings, and smell to create a desired state in her mind. These were used in combination with relaxation and deep breathing to produce stress reduction when she was faced with daily pressures.

This mind/body tool has been used as part of the treatment for anxiety. For people with anxiety disorders, medications and psychotherapy are important treatments. If visualization does not reduce symptoms, it's important to get additional help from a physician or licensed mental-health professional.

In the past few years the connection between imagery and the immune system has been studied frequently. In 1980 Simonton and Sparks used imagery as intervention for clients with advanced cancer. In comparing their study with nationally established survival rates for breast, colon, and lung cancer, the researchers found that clients who practiced imagery in combination with traditional medical treatment had a prolonged life expectancy. Another study in 1988 by Benson and colleagues reported that patients who practiced imagery with relaxation felt less emotional distress and reported decreased nausea and vomiting following chemotherapy.

If you have trouble imagining scenes and images to de-stress, listen to sounds of waves or thunderstorms to trigger thoughts of natural settings. Relaxation tapes and CDs with nature sounds can be purchased at any music store.

YOGA OR TAI CHI

There are many ways to infuse a sense of calmness into a hectic day to curb stress eating, and for many people, yoga or tai chi is part of their answer. Yoga is an old Hindu technique using deep breathing, concentration techniques, and body poses to calm your mind and improve flexibility. Tai chi is a Chinese art focusing on balance and coordination from gentle, graceful movements along with breathing, patterns that may lower blood pressure and heart rate.

Both of these ancient disciplines are easy to learn, don't require you to invest a fortune on equipment, and work for almost any physical activity level. The few studies that have been done evaluating their effects point to improvement in mood. Yoga is recommended by author Dean Ornish, M.D., in his program of creative lifestyle changes for patients with coronary heart disease. Whether or not it prevents or treats disease may not be certain, but both yoga and tai chi have an ability to calm and relax you.

Although there are no licensing standards for yoga or tai chi instructors, several organizations do train and certify teachers. Talk to friends who have learned these disciplines, talk to the instructor, and sit through a class before making a commitment.

DEEP ABDOMINAL BREATHING

Remember Elizabeth, the young woman who had great difficulty reacting under pressure? After learning guided imagery, she became an avid believer in adding deep breathing to reduce perceived stress. She found that breathing can measure and alter her psychological state, making a stressful moment accelerate or diminish in intensity. "I used to take breathing for granted," she told us confidently. "But I've started tuning in to my body before a presentation at work or when I'm up against a deadline. I found that my respiration was quickening because of my anxiety and fear, which seemed to trigger the stress response. I've now mastered this deep-breathing technique and use deep, slow breaths for a calming effect."

Breathing is an involuntary activity of the body that people can consciously control. Before a presentation to a large group of people or a television show, we both use this mind/body tool to de-stress. As you learn how to do deep abdominal breathing, you will gain control over a basic physiological function, helping to decrease the release of stress hormones, and slow down your heartbeat during stressful moments.

MASSAGE

Who wouldn't agree that getting a massage feels great? There is some new evidence that touching not only feels good, it also promotes healing. Called massage by most and positive structured touch (PST) by others, both manual and mechanical massage seem to make a difference in recovery from fatigue after exercise. It is reported that an estimated 30,000 North American nurses employ therapeutic touch. In fact, studies released from the University of Miami School of Medicine's Touch Research Center found that the benefits of massage include heightened alertness, relief from depression and anxiety, an increase in the number of natural "killer cells" in the immune system, lower levels of the stress hormone cortisol, and reduced difficulty in getting to sleep.

There are many types of massage, but Swedish is the most common, using long, kneading strokes and gentle vibrations to relax the superficial muscle layers. In Japanese, shiatsu or "finger pressure" is a technique that uses acupressure to specific points on the body. Pressure may be applied by fingers, thumbs, even elbows and knees. The American Massage Therapy Association provides a national referral service for qualified, professional massage therapists.

PROGRESSIVE MUSCLE RELAXATION

This exercise is also known as deep muscle relaxation. It involves concentrating on different muscle groups as you contract then relax all of the major muscle groups in the body, beginning with head, neck, arms, chest, back, stomach, pelvis, legs, and feet. As you will learn in Stress-Less Strategy #3, to do this exercise, you will focus on each set of muscles, tense these muscles to the count of ten, then release to the count of ten. Along with progressive muscle relaxation, it is important to perform the deep abdominal breathing, breathing in while tensing the muscles, and breathing out or exhaling while relaxing them.

BIOFEEDBACK

If after trying some of the mind/body techniques in this chapter you are still having trouble calming down from daily stress, you may want to look into biofeedback. This relaxation technique is based on the theory that you can learn to control to some degree responses that are considered involuntary such as heart rate and blood pressure. By placing electric sensors on the body, data on body temperature, respiration, or muscle tension can be sent to a monitor as you react to various stimuli such as thoughts, pictures, or sounds. By studying the body's reactions to these stimuli, a person can be taught to recognize feelings of tension and learn methods to calm him- or herself. Although there is controversy about the effectiveness of biofeedback for some illnesses, the technique is used by many psychologists and stress-management professionals. This skill of relaxing is then used outside the therapist's office when you encounter the day-to-day stresses of life. Some therapists recommend relaxation tapes that can be listened to at home to practice relaxation techniques.

The main concept is centered around the idea that you may not be able to control what goes on around you, but you can learn to alter the way you respond to it.

LAUGHTER THERAPY

We both enjoy a good laugh. In fact, there were times when we were burning the midnight oil while doing research for *I'd Kill for a Cookie* that we would close the books and sit down with a bowl of popcorn to catch a rerun of *Seinfeld* or *I Love Lucy*. To us, laughter is great medicine for our busy minds and stressed bodies.

We're sure that it is no news to you that laughing can help you unwind, unless you are like Harold. This forty-seven-year-old hospital administrator came to learn how the EAT Plan could help him de-stress. Harold carried the worries of the world on his shoulders, and with each new problem at the hospital, his blood pressure jumped another five points. "Laugh?" Harold acted surprised. "I can't remember the last time I really laughed. My life just isn't funny."

We reminded this serious businessman how for centuries, humor and health have been closely tied together. Even in biblical times, writers reported that "a merry heart doeth good like a medicine" (Proverbs 17:22). Instead of receiving a "how-to" list of things to do to unwind, we told Harold to start by renting some funny videos and making a commitment for three weeks to "turn off" his work problems when he got home. He took our advice to heart, and instead of dwelling on how to make a profit, he focused instead on the humor in the movies. Not surprisingly, after a few weeks of doing this consistently, this once-somber man had lightened up a bit and was realizing the benefits with less stress symptoms, reduced blood pressure, and a new zest for life.

Remember, your brain will only react to what you feed it. When your boss reprimands you or you find that your two-year-old has stripped the wallpaper in his room, you send negative distress signals to your brain. The brain will react by signaling the fight-or-flight response to every organ in the body. Here goes the red alert! Yet you can learn to send positive signals, even when you are facing stress, and your brain will react with a sense of support and solidarity, causing physiological changes that are healing. (Note: Please don't laugh in your boss's face or when your child is being destructive or disobedient. Wait until you've left the room, and let it roll.)

Researchers are finding that laughing has an added bonus as it seems to strengthen the immune system. Some studies have shown that people who laugh hard produce more immunoglobulin A, which strengthens your ability to fight infection. Your heart rate increases, the oxygen to the brain is boosted, and your blood flow improves. When you relax afterwards, your body calms down.

Duke University began a humor project in 1988 with its Laugh Mobile, which employees rolled from room to room to provide comic relief with items like funny movies, bottles of bubble soap, Nerf balls, and comic books. More recently, Dr. John Graham-Pole, who runs the bone marrow transplant unit at Shands Hospital in Gainesville, Florida, has taken humor and healing seriously. After spending much time searching for a connection between the body and mind, this innovative physician found that the use of laughter, clowning, and poetry with his oncology patients and staff members brought a healing atmosphere. Inspired by Graham-Pole's actions, Shands now has an Arts in Medicine program with a creative staff comprised of a dancer, a painter, a writer, a sculptor, and two guitarists—all to help patients express their emotions about their illness and treatment.

IT'S TIME FOR HEALING

The EAT Plan will help you put your life in perspective as you start to focus on activity as something that you do for play—yes, we want you to enjoy this—instead of viewing exercise as punishment. We have found that often attitudes need healing as much as the body, and looking at the whole person is very important. You can find humor in the midst of stress. This is when you really need it and when your sense of humor usually abandons you.

The longer the two of us live, the more we realize the impact of attitude in our lives. Even though we went to school for years to learn the latest in scientific theory, we have found attitude to be at least as important to us as fact. We know that our attitude can make or break our success and happiness in life. What is most remarkable is that we have the choice every day regarding the attitude we will embrace.

We cannot change our past; you cannot change yours. How you responded to stress yesterday is history. But we do know that you can change your attitude and how you respond to stress right now, tomorrow, and in the days to come. We know that with the EAT Plan, you can follow in the successful footsteps of others before you as you learn, once and for all, how to conquer stress and the resulting stress eating.

Are you ready to make some attitude adjustments? We hope so, for it is now time to make some positive lifestyle changes with six stress-less strategies that can change your life forever. Good luck!

c h a p t e r   6

———◆———

STOP STRESS EATING NOW
WITH THE EAT PLAN

Now that you understand the reasons for the EAT Plan, you are ready to start making positive changes to conquer stress eating. The EAT Plan is your Energy-Action Team. Over the next six weeks, this team approach will work with your strengths and fill in where problems exist so you can make the stress in your life work with you instead of against you.

Your Energy-Action Team consists of six stress-less strategies, one for each week. You will learn to:

1. Eat to combat stress and boost immunity;
2. Eat to enhance your mood;
3. Move to create happy hormones;
4. Plan your time and prioritize;
5. Revamp your pantry; and
6. Hit the road running.

While each of these members of the team is equally important, you can start with any one of them. However we recommend starting week one with Stress-Less Strategy #1 so you can begin to shake the negative effects of stress right away while you work with the other members of the team. Although it will take time to make the changes you desire in your lifestyle, progress through strategies 2 to 6 over the next five weeks so that your entire plan is put into action. Then you can continue to fine-tune each strategy that needs extra attention until you no longer want to kill for a cookie.

STRESS-LESS STRATEGY #1: CAPTURE THE POWER OF ANTIOXIDANTS AND PHYTOCHEMICALS

It is the first week of your EAT Plan, and we know that you are anxious to finally start doing something healthful for your body. This week you will learn to implement Stress-Less Strategy #1, which is to combat stress and boost immunity by choosing foods high in phytochemicals and antioxidants (vitamin C, vitamin E, and the carotenoids including beta-carotene).

You already know the immune-boosting benefits of eating these foods (see pages 27 to 29), so let's begin to incorporate these phytochemicals and antioxidants into your daily diet so that you will be in better shape to cope with the effects of stress, whether physical or emotional.

STEP #1: EAT MORE ANTIOXIDANT FRUITS AND VEGETABLES

"My mother always told me to eat fruits and vegetables. I honestly never thought there was a reason behind it." Cindy, a self-proclaimed "junk food junkie," came to see us for help with boosting her energy level to handle her new stressful sales job and was surprised when we pulled out the chart of phytochemicals that are essential to our EAT Plan.

What Cindy didn't realize is that since her childhood days and in particular just recently researchers have uncovered new and potentially more important reasons to eat fruits and vegetables. While these foods are loaded with vitamins, minerals, and fiber and have little or no fat, that's only half the story.

Experts estimate that eating a "junk food diet" like Cindy's is responsible for anywhere from 10 to 70 percent of all cancers; in fact, most researchers would say it is much closer to 70 percent than 10 percent. While much of the focus for disease prevention used to be on lowering the fat in the diet, one opinion is that the benefit of a low-fat diet may be more from what you *do eat* than from what you leave out. That is, the newest and most important benefits to wellness and the stress-disease connection are the antioxidant and phytochemical content of these foods.

Immune System under Fire

From a stress standpoint, we know the immune system is brutally challenged under stress. Under stress, the body doesn't need the mechanisms that will fight infection in the future or protect our cells from cancer or heart disease. Rather, it needs to get ready for the fight-or-flight response pronto, so we can escape the stressor. Antioxidants work to boost immune function during and after stress, and while the immune system may not achieve a pre-stress level, antioxidants will undo some of the damage caused by stress.

To explain the antioxidant effect, think of your body as your car. Every day it is exposed to air, humidity, and sometimes rain, snow, or even hail. If not protected, over a period of time your car will develop rust. Rust can be compared to the free-radical buildup that humans also get over time, especially as added stress reduces our immunity. Antioxidants act as a protective shield for our cells, keeping them from the harmful effects of free radicals. This is like purchasing a rust coating to protect your car, except all you have to do is eat fruits and vegetables.

The unfortunate fact is that most people don't take advantage of this breakthrough information. The United States Department of Agriculture (USDA) reported recently that only about 9 percent of Americans eat the recommended five servings of fruits and vegetables every day. We honestly believe that you can do even better. Researchers for the National Cancer Institute would like all of us to aim even higher, to nine fruits and vegetables each day. A serving is smaller than you may expect. For example, four ounces of orange juice is equal to one serving as is one half cup of broccoli or one half of a banana. So eat the whole banana, and you are well on your way to five servings a day.

Look how easy it is to accumulate five servings in one day:

Breakfast	8 oz. orange juice (1)* and (2)*
	cereal and milk
Lunch:	turkey sandwich
	chips
	apple (3)*
Dinner:	baked chicken
	rice
	1 cup broccoli (4)* and (5)*
	frozen yogurt

* = Servings

While it may take a little planning and focusing on these foods, it does not take much more effort to get the protective benefit of nine servings. Add to breakfast: 1 banana on the cereal (6)* and (7)*. Add to dinner: 1 cup of spinach or romaine lettuce salad (8)* and (9)*.

Protect Yourself and Your Family

The problem with adding more fruits and vegetables to the diet is that these habits must start young, and most of us still think that ketchup and french fries count as vegetables for the day. It's interesting that a group of kindergartners observed by Michigan State University researchers said the "grossest foods" are tomatoes, olives, mushrooms, broccoli, brussels sprouts, potatoes, and potato salad. Favorite foods listed were pizza, macaroni and cheese, meat, eggs, and ice cream. The frightening news is that the favorite foods of these five-year-olds are some of the lowest in antioxidants. Our job, should we choose to accept it, is to find new and exciting ways to eat our veggies.

Here is a list of the top ten food sources of antioxidants:

1. Broccoli
2. Cantaloupe
3. Papaya
4. Spinach
5. Brussels sprouts
6. Asparagus
7. Carrots
8. Tomatoes
9. Peaches
10. Nectarines

CHECK YOUR LOCAL FARMERS' MARKET

Local farmers' markets are a great place to stock up on fruits and vegetables. You can get a complete list of farmers' markets by writing to the USDA, P.O. Box 96456, Room 2642 South, Washington, D.C. 20090.

The Most Common Antioxidants

The antioxidant nutrients most readily available from food include vitamin C, vitamin E, and the carotenoids, which include beta-carotene.

Vitamin E. Some of the most encouraging reports about vitamin E have been studies that looked at the effects of the nutrient in levels not often found in everyday diets. Since vitamin E is found in vegetable and seed oils, it is hard to get large amounts from food and still maintain a diet low in fat. In fact, we do not need to restrict fat as severely as many have if the fat we eat is from plant oils that are monounsaturated like olive oil, canola oil, and peanut oil. Studies have shown reduced heart disease and cancer risk in populations using these oils as their primary fat source. Still, many people are looking at vitamin E supplements as extra protection.

HOW MUCH IS ENOUGH?

If you decide to take a supplement, you need relatively low doses, 130 to 260 milligrams (200 to 400 IU) daily to achieve the benefit found in clinical studies.

Vitamin C. This nutrient is readily available in fruits and vegetables. It is destroyed by heat, so raw is best, but a short cooking time in a small amount of water also preserves the nutrient. This one is easy to get through food.

Start your day with orange or grapefruit juice, put a slice or two of tomato on your sandwich at lunch, then have some broccoli at dinner, and you've substantially added to your antioxidant total for the day. In fact, with just those three foods, you have tripled the amount of vitamin C required to prevent a deficiency.

The latest research is indicating that preventing deficiency is not our only goal with these nutrients. Especially when under stress, we need to maximize the protective effect of antioxidants and reach for more than the amount designed to prevent deficiency. Vitamin C is depleted during stress so to combat it, we need to focus on many and varied food sources.

FOODS RICH IN VITAMIN C

Broccoli	Papayas
Cabbage	Passion fruit
Carambola or star fruit	Pomelos
Citrus fruits	Potatoes
Green peppers	Strawberries
Mangoes	Tomatoes

Vitamin C in a Pill?

Supplements up to 1,500 milligrams daily can be used without harm for people who don't eat many fruits and vegetables, but we want to draw your attention to some cautions. First, chewable vitamin C wears down tooth enamel. It is an acid, after all (ascorbic acid is the chemical name for vitamin C). If you want to take supplements, opt for swallowable rather than the chewable variety. Second, all you get in the pill is vitamin C. If you are not eating fruits and vegetables, you are missing the fiber, other nutrients, and the whole array of phytochemicals we'll discuss next.

We take vitamin C supplements when we travel and when our stress levels are high. They may also help in the earliest stage of a cold to combat symptoms, as vitamin C mimics the effect of an antihistamine.

During periods when you crave fruits and vegetables because you haven't had your usual quota, a supplement can be a temporary insurance policy until you get back on the produce wagon. Buy the generic brands that are less expensive, because you don't need chelated or other supposed benefits. Split your dose and take vitamin C morning and night to maintain constant blood levels over a twenty-four-hour period.

Carotenoids. The third member of the antioxidant team, the carotenoids, come from yellow, orange, or red fruits and vegetables or green leafy vegetables. Most people have focused all their interest on beta-carotene as having antioxidant properties, but there are many other carotenoid compounds that are also beneficial.

Carotenoid	Food Source
Alpha-carotene	Carrots, cantaloupe, guava, pumpkin, yellow corn
Beta-carotene	Apricots, carrots, cantaloupe, pumpkin, spinach and other leafy greens, sweet potatoes
Gamma-carotene	Apricots, tomatoes

Carotenoid	Food Source
Beta-cryptoxanthin	Mangoes, nectarines, oranges, papayas, peaches, tangerines
Lycopene	Guava, pink grapefruit, tomatoes, watermelon
Lutein, zeaxanthin	Beets, collard and mustard greens, chicory, chili peppers, corn, kale, spinach

STEP #2: EAT MORE PHYTOCHEMICAL FRUITS, VEGETABLES, AND GRAINS

"Phyto-what? Why do I need to eat something that I can't even say?" Remember Cindy, the "junk-food junkie?" Her ears really perked up when we began telling her about phytochemicals and how these are necessary for immune power in addition to the antioxidants in fruits and vegetables. Researchers have uncovered another group of chemicals found naturally in plant foods that are working hard to guard and improve our health. These chemicals are now called phyto-chemicals, phytonutrients, or phytomedicine. It is believed that in nature phytochemicals help protect the plant from harmful effects of its environment. There are probably hundreds of different phytochemi-cals, and each fruit, vegetable, or grain contains its own unique mix.

Let's take a quick look at some of them and what they do for you.

The Lowdown on Phytochemicals

Phytochemical	Food Sources	Health Effect
Sulfides (allyl)	Garlic, onions, cabbage, broccoli, brussels sprouts	Cancer prevention, suppress tumor development
Capsaicin	Hot chili peppers, Thai peppers, jalapenos	Cancer prevention
Carotenoids	Carrots, winter squash, sweet potatoes, apricots, spinach, kale, parsley, soybeans, cereal grains	Antioxidant, heart disease and cancer prevention, and improved immune function

Phytochemical	Food Sources	Health Effect
Bioflavonoids	Most vegetables and fruits, licorice, flax seed, green tea	Cancer prevention
Ellagic acid	Grapes, apples, strawberries, raspberries	Heart disease and cancer prevention
Isoflavones	Soybeans, legumes	Cancer prevention and menopause symptom reduction
Indoles	Cruciferous vegetables such as cauliflower, broccoli, brussels sprouts, cabbage, bok choy, kale, mustard seed, radishes	Cancer prevention
Isothiocyanates	Mustard, radishes, horseradish	Cancer prevention
Limonoids, terpenes	All citrus fruits	Cancer prevention
Linolenic Acid	Leafy vegetables, seeds, flax seed	Heart disease and cancer prevention
Lycopene	Tomatoes, watermelon, pink grapefruit, guava, red peppers	Cancer prevention
Monoterpenes	Garlic, parsley, squash, basil, mint, eggplant, citrus, tomatoes	Antioxidant, heart disease and cancer prevention
Phenolic acids	Garlic, green tea, cereal grains, soybeans, fruits, vegetables, licorice root, flax seed	Antioxidant, heart disease and cancer prevention

Phytochemical	Food Sources	Health Effect
Plant sterols	Broccoli, cabbage, soy products, peppers, whole grains	Cancer prevention
Sulforaphane	Broccoli, cabbage, cauliflower, onions, brussels sprouts	Cancer prevention

Ways to Add Phytochemicals

Instead of:	Use:
Iceberg lettuce	Romaine, spinach, red or green leaf
Tomato sauce	Vegetable sauce (add shredded carrots or zucchini)
White grapefruit	Pink grapefruit
Cole slaw	Broccoslaw (bagged in the produce section)
White potatoes	Sweet potatoes
Hamburger	Tofu crumbles, soy burgers, or portabello mushrooms
Sausage	Soy-based sausage
Chili con carne	Meatless chili with beans or tofu

The Benefits of Soy

Most people eat very little in the way of soy foods, yet even adding one serving a day can make a dramatic difference in reducing the risk of disease.

Isoflavones. Two components of the common soybean, daidzein and genistein, have been shown to have beneficial effects in cancer prevention and the prevention of heart disease and osteoporosis, along with reducing the symptoms of menopause. Genistein can help prevent breast cancer by blocking the receptors for estrogen on breast cells and preventing estrogen from promoting tumor growth. The anti-cancer effect is not limited to breast cancer alone. Other cancers that are not estrogen dependent also respond to genistein because it limits the enzymes that convert normal cells to cancer cells.

In the area of heart disease, eating soy protein lowers cholesterol, particularly the LDL cholesterol that is associated with increased heart disease risk. In osteoporosis research, daidzein and genistein have been shown to inhibit bone breakdown in animals. Eating soy protein also causes less calcium loss in the urine than animal protein, thus keeping bones' calcium dense and strong.

Use the following soy foods that are already available, and watch for new food products as the interest in soy for health expands:

- Soy milk: Use this on cereal, in baking when milk is called for, and in milk shakes or Phyto-Fruit Smoothies (see pages 130–132). We like the vanilla-flavored soy milk. Look for calcium-fortified soy milk so the calcium content will be similar to that of regular milk.
- Tofu: Silken tofu works well in shakes, puddings, or soups for a creamy texture. Tofu can also be used as a meat substitute; use tofu crumbles in chili, tacos, or sloppy joe sandwiches.
- Use the soy-substitute burgers, sausages, or bacon, and crumbles instead of meat in your favorite recipes.
- Soy flour: Substitute about one-quarter of the flour in baking recipes with soy flour.
- Soybeans: Dried beans can be used in recipes such as baked beans or chili. Remember to soak them first, like any dried bean.

STEP #3: REVIEW YOUR NEED FOR SUPPLEMENTS

Now that we know the benefits of these foods, supplement manufacturers are hot on the trail of, you guessed it, vegetable supplements. A trip to your local health-food store or pharmacy can be like visiting the produce market, except in pill form. You don't have to look very long before you'll discover broccoli pills, garlic pills, spinach pills, and various "mixed vegetable" pills. These are marketed for people who don't like vegetables, or who are afraid they don't eat enough vegetables so they want to supplement with a pill. One problem with this approach is that we are in the preliminary stages of identifying these important chemicals so the pills don't contain them all, and the amount in a pill may not even be close to what you would get if you ate the foods. Realistically, even if they develop a pill for every phytochemical identified, you would end up taking forty to sixty pills a day to get the same effect of eating fruits and vegetables. Vegetable pills won't hurt you, but we don't have data to tell us they can help you either.

You may be wondering, Why don't we just eat the phyto-loaded vegetables and fruits we like? Simple enough! For example, if you eat spinach, you get the whole package, including the fiber, and other nutrients like vitamin C. The whole vegetable includes all of the substances we know to be beneficial and probably some we don't know about yet.

Tip #1: Some supplements may be necessary. For years we have been encouraging people to improve their diets so they can get all the nutrients they need through food. This is smart advice, especially since there are now some newly identified substances in food that may actually prevent disease. However, the problem is that most people don't eat fruits and vegetables in the quantities recommended. While we agree with the goal of increasing fruit and vegetable consumption and aim for five to nine servings of fruits and vegetables a day ourselves, supplements can be a fairly cheap insurance policy for getting part of what you need while you work on improving your diet. And remember, when we are under stress, our diets usually get worse, not better.

RECOMMENDED VITAMIN SUPPLEMENTS*

- Start with a multivitamin without minerals as a basic supplement. (The B vitamins are covered by this multivitamin.)
- Add iron as needed. Check with your health care professional. Men and postmenopausal women do not need extra iron.
- Add 500 milligrams vitamin C daily. If you are under stress or getting a cold, take 1,000 to 2,000 milligrams daily for a week or less.
- Add 200 to 400 IU vitamin E daily.
- Add calcium supplements of 500 to 1,500 milligrams daily, depending on your food intake of calcium-rich foods and your age. One cup of milk contains about 300 milligrams of calcium, as does $1^{1}/_{2}$ ounces of cheddar cheese or $^{3}/_{4}$ cup of plain yogurt. Premenopausal women should aim for 1,000 milligrams a day. Postmenopausal women who don't take estrogen replacement need 1,500 milligrams a day.
- Add vitamin D (400 IU) if your vitamin D intake is low or sun exposure is limited. Many older people do not get enough vitamin D, especially in the winter months when days are shorter and sunshine is limited.
- Add up to 15 milligrams (or 25,000 IU) beta-carotene when fruit and vegetable intake is below five servings per day.

Consult with an R.D. (registered dietitian) for a complete nutrition checkup, if you think you need more vitamins or have questions.

MAJOR SOURCES OF VITAMIN D

Milk

Fatty fish (such as salmon, herring, mackerel or sardines)

Fortified cereals

Sunshine exposure

1 milligram beta-carotene = 1,675 IU

PRIMARY FOOD SOURCES OF CALCIUM

Milk and milk products

Dark, green leafy vegetables

Calcium-fortified juices and breads

Canned salmon (including the bones)

A WORD ON CALCIUM SUPPLEMENTS

- Look for supplements in the form of calcium carbonate or calcium citrate.
- Calcium carbonate should be taken with food to increase absorption.
- Take calcium in divided doses with the last dose at bedtime.
- If you drink skim milk, try adding $\frac{1}{4}$ cup dry milk to each cup of skim to double your calcium.

TAKE THE VINEGAR TEST

Do you wonder if your vitamin supplement is being absorbed by your body? Drop samples of your vitamin tablets in a glass filled with two inches of vinegar. Leave them for thirty to forty-five minutes. If the vitamins dissolve, they should be absorbed in your body. But if after forty-five minutes your vitamins stay intact, you may as well toss the bottles away, for the likelihood is they are not being absorbed in your body.

PHYTOCHEMICAL MENUS

Here are some easy and quick ways to boost these stress-fighting chemicals in your daily eating.

BREAKFAST

- Fruit or vegetable juices (grab the cans and drink on the way)
- Melon
- Grapefruit or pineapple (buy sectioned in the produce department)
- Soy milk on cereal
- Soy flour in quick breads like banana or zucchini bread
- Soy sausage patties or soy bacon strips
- Citrus friut
- Other fruit

LUNCH
<ul><li>Salads with romaine, spinach, green- or red-leaf lettuce as the main ingredient</li><li>Veggie sandwiches</li><li>Portabello mushroom burgers</li><li>Baked potatoes with salsa or chili topping</li><li>Vegetable soups</li><li>Tabbouleh pita pockets</li><li>Tomatoes added to sandwiches</li><li>Chinese vegetables over rice</li><li>Bean burritos</li><li>Chili with beans or soy protein</li></ul>

DINNER
<ul><li>Same as lunch plus bagged salads from the produce department, and lots of veggies, fresh, frozen, or canned.</li></ul>

SNACKS
<ul><li>Fresh fruit (don't forget tropical fruits like mangoes, kiwi, pineapple) dried fruits like apricots, cherries, cranberries, or sun-dried strawberries</li><li>Carrots in a bag from the produce department</li><li>Broccoli or cauliflower with ranch dip</li><li>Phyto-Fruit Smoothies</li></ul>

Recipe for Phyto-Fruit Smoothies

We know that too much stress can zap you of energy, and usually at the worst times. The EAT Plan is about prevention—preventing stress from taking over your life and your health by nourishing and healing your body with phytonutrients. Enjoy the following fruit smoothies any time you need a quick pick-me-up, especially when you are feeling bummed out from too much stress. Using a blender or food processor, mix up a batch of your favorite flavors, blend thoroughly, and enjoy the added benefit of good health and stress protection.

For yogurt, use plain, non-fat, low-fat, frozen, or flavored—your choice! For variation, add 2 tablespoons of wheat germ, 2 tablespoons of chocolate syrup, or flavorings like vanilla, peppermint, rum, or lemon.

Berry-Banana Cooler: 1 cup strawberries or mixed berries, 1 banana, 1 cup low-fat vanilla frozen yogurt, and 5–6 cubes of ice.

Mango Mania: One cup mango, 1 banana, 1 cup pineapple sherbet, and ice.

Banana Split: One cup skim milk, $1/2$ cup strawberries, 3 tablespoons chocolate syrup, 1 banana, 1 cup low-fat vanilla yogurt, and ice.

Creamsicle: One cup orange juice, 1 banana, 1 cup vanilla low-fat yogurt, and ice.

PB&J: 1 cup apple juice, 2 tablespoons peanut butter, $1/2$ cup strawberries, 1 banana, 1 cup low-fat vanilla yogurt, and ice.

Lemon Squeezer: One cup berries, 1 banana, $1/2$ cup low-fat vanilla frozen yogurt, $1/2$ cup lemon sherbet, and ice.

Piña-Coolada; $1/2$ cup pineapple juice, $1/4$ cup shredded coconut, 1 banana, 1 cup low-fat vanilla frozen yogurt, and ice.

Peach Melba: $1/2$ cup sliced peaches, $1/2$ cup raspberries, 1 banana, 1 cup raspberry sherbet, and ice.

Lime-onade: 2 tablespoons limeade, 2 teaspoons lemon

juice, 2 teaspoons honey, 1 banana, $^1/_2$ cup low-fat vanilla frozen yogurt, $^1/_2$ cup lemon or lime sherbet, and ice.

Nut Case: 2 tablespoons peanut butter, 2 tablespoons chocolate syrup, 1 banana, 1 cup low-fat vanilla frozen yogurt, and ice.

Ship-a-soy: $^1/_2$ cup light soy milk, 1 cup low-fat vanilla yogurt, 3–4 tablespoons frozen orange juice concentrate (unthawed), 1 banana, 2 tablespoons wheat germ. Add ice if a frozen consistency is desired.

CHECKLIST FOR STRESS-LESS STRATEGY #1

_____ Eat more antioxidant fruits and vegetables.
_____ Eat more phytochemical fruits, vegetables, and grains.
_____ Review your need for supplements.

STRESS-LESS STRATEGY #2: BECOME AN ACTIVE MOOD MANAGER

Perhaps as you have been reading *I'd Kill for a Cookie*, you have dreamed of being more alert and productive all day long, yet your caffeine habit does not seem to give you the mental boost you need. What about anxiety? Do you often feel the signs of too much stress? Are you often too keyed up at night to rest and need some workable tips on how to get healing sleep? Then keep reading, for week #2 will start you on the road to becoming an Active Mood Manager as you learn some winning techniques that can change the way you feel all day long.

The research on the food-mood connection has come a long way since our childhood days when Popeye relied on spinach for strength and energy. Using the latest breakthrough findings, this stress-less strategy will help you to chart a road map for success as you rearrange your eating for maximum productivity and manipulate your circadian clock to work for you.

"How can changing what I eat or when I eat make me more productive? I barely have time to make sure my kids are fed, let alone myself," Jane, a stay-at-home mom with three preschoolers, complained. We explained that research is continually exploring the complex relationships between food, mood, and performance. You read examples of some of these studies in Chapter 4, and now it's time to put those principles to work.

STEP #1: TAKE YOUR PERSONAL FOOD BAROMETER

Using the following Food Barometer, write down your specific food-mood response after eating. A sample is given for you.

Sample Personal Food Barometer

Day	Time	Food	Mood Response
Mon.	7:00 A.M.	Grilled cheese	More alert than usual
Mon.	12:30 P.M.	Pasta salad, bread	Sleepy time after lunch
Mon.	4:00 P.M.	Low-fat cheese	Felt energetic, did not overeat later
Mon.	7:00 P.M.	Roast chicken, rice, broccoli	Alert; paid bills
Tues.	7:00 A.M.	Banana, juice	Needed java at work to wake up
Tues.	12:00 P.M.	Ham and cheese sandwich	Finished big project at work
Tues.	6:15 P.M.	Macaroni, veggies, ice milk	Slept like a baby—went to bed early
Wed.	7:00 A.M.	Scrambled egg w/cheese	Felt great giving my presentation
Wed.	1:00 P.M.	Bagel and cream cheese	Tired and sleepy

Day	Time	Food	Mood Response
Wed.	7:00 P.M.	Client dinner—lobster & filet	New contract very possible!

Personal Food Barometer Work Sheet

Day	Time	Food	Mood Response
___	___	___	___
___	___	___	___
___	___	___	___
___	___	___	___
___	___	___	___
___	___	___	___
___	___	___	___
___	___	___	___
___	___	___	___
___	___	___	___

STEP #2: USE FOOD TO HELP YOUR MOOD

Research studies continue to divulge information on how the foods we eat affect our moods and activity level. We discussed the latest research by Dr. Judith Wurtman in Chapter 4. Another closely related study yielded the same results as Dr. Wurtman's. Drs. Madelyn Fernstrom and John Fernstrom at the University of Pittsburgh found that in animals, meals containing carbohydrate versus protein had different mood effects, and the moods changed when the next meal was eaten. To put this research in human terms: If we load up on carbohydrates for lunch (such as pasta with tomato sauce, bread, and salad), the neurotransmitter serotonin is increased; we may feel drowsy and less alert for the next two to three hours. If we then have grilled chicken and vegetables for dinner, the neurotransmitters dopamine and norepinephrine will increase; the drowsiness effect will be reversed. When the protein meal was fed first, eating carbohydrates at least three hours later caused a change in serotonin levels.

There is still much controversy as to the extent that these animal studies reflect what happens in humans. However, it is important to recognize that there is little disagreement from the human studies; that is, in distressed people, there is a definite link between food and mood.

Here are tips to guide you in becoming your own Active Mood Manager:

Tip #1: Try high-protein foods to boost alertness. Now that you have completed the Personal Food Barometer (Step #1), it is time to use this information to boost your alertness when needed. Incorporate some low-fat protein foods into your day when you need a lift or feel generally tired or sluggish.

Top Ten Energy Boosters

1. Shellfish and fish (except salmon, mackerel, and any thing fried)
2. Chicken (baked, roasted, broiled, steamed, poached, or stewed, sliced as deli meat, or ground)
3. Turkey (same as above)
4. Lean ham or pork tenderloin
5. Lean beef such as flank steak, London broil, or filet mignon
6. Skim milk
7. Low-fat yogurt
8. Low-fat or no-fat cheese
9. Beans and peas
10. Soy milk and tofu

Tip #2: Use serotonin-boosting carbohydrates to relax and calm down. Review your response to the Personal Food Barometer, and see if the following top ten relaxation foods can help you to de-stress.

Top Ten Relaxation Foods

1. Cookies
2. Breads
3. Pasta
4. Rice, couscous, corn, or other grains
5. Popcorn
6. Crackers
7. Potatoes
8. Cereals
9. Chocolate
10. Other sweets

Tip #3: Keep in mind that the food/mood reaction is short-term. "All right, now that I know how food influences my moods and energy level, I can change the way I eat," Margie, a public relations executive, told us. "If I need to feel alert all day for a seminar, I should eat eggs for breakfast." Margie was correct in that the protein in eggs for breakfast will help to jump-start alertness and energy, but she will need to throw in a high-protein snack and lunch as well, to continue this mood-boosting response.

Research has shown that these effects of certain foods on mood are not long-lasting. For example, the effect of a food such as tuna fish will cause an increased alertness for up to two to three hours after the meal, not for days or weeks. Also, the serotonin response, that is, foods giving a calming effect, seems to last up to two to three hours after a carbohydrate meal, such as pancakes with syrup. Because of this short-term effect of food on mood, we have established grazing or eating mini-meals within our EAT Plan that will help you use this food-mood connection to your advantage. You will learn how to do this in Stress-Less Strategy #4.

Tip #4: Monitor portion size for calming down or boosting energy. For those who need to relax or calm down after a stressful day, we have found that even small portions of serotonin-boosting foods can make a difference. Try one ounce of chocolate, two cookies, a cup of cereal or pasta or two slices of bread to feel calmer. (Don't eat all of these at once. Yes, you may feel calm, but you may also gain weight!)

For those who feel lackadaisical and just cannot get moving, you can try two ounces of lean meat or cheese or $1\frac{1}{2}$ cups of milk, yogurt, or beans to get an energy boost. Dr. Wurtman suggests eating low-fat, high-protein foods for lunch to achieve maximum afternoon alertness. Try tuna or turkey on whole wheat bread with fruit salad; low-fat yogurt or cottage cheese, and a whole-wheat roll; or thin-crust pizza with veggies and low-fat cheese. Cathy finds that salad with grilled chicken breast helps to keep her alert on busy seminar days, while Susan grazes on string cheese and crackers during her heavy teaching schedule. Many of our clients have also successfully used protein foods throughout their busy days and found increased mental alertness.

Tip #5: Understand your brain chemistry. How does our brain chemistry relate to what we eat and feel? Research at Rockefeller University in New York suggests that at different times of the day, certain brain chemicals are more prevalent. Sarah Leibowitz, a neurobiologist at Rockefeller University, has been studying the link between brain chemistry and appetite for more than fifteen years and has found that these varying brain chemicals are behind the reasons we want certain foods at different meals. For example, in animal studies a chemical called neuropeptide Y (NPY) and the hormone cortisol are found in high levels in the brain in the mornings and seem to increase the desire for carbohydrates. This might explain why you reach for an English muffin or crunchy cereal instead of cheese pizza or your favorite burger.

Serotonin is produced as those carbohydrates are digested. Serotonin signals the shutoff of NPY, and as lunchtime approaches, the brain wants protein. Could that be why a turkey sandwich with Swiss looks so good? The next neurochemical, called galanin, takes the lead and appears to whet our desire for fat. Rich, fatty foods are the focus for many in the afternoon and on into the evening.

According to Leibowitz, this is a normal pattern of the body because first thing in the morning, the blood glucose (blood sugar) level is low and the muscle fuel, or glycogen, is depleted. Carbohydrates are a quick energy source, so it seems natural to reach for them. As your day goes on and your body is working as a finely tuned machine (or will be after you finished the EAT Plan), protein is needed to build muscle, for maintenance and repair. Leibowitz indicates that our desire for fat at night is due to the body's need to deposit reserves for overnight hibernation.

When we were children, these fat cravings were not a strong force. But for most women of childbearing age, this is an important tip tied to menstruation. Have you ever noticed that certain times during your cycle as well as the time of day can affect your desire for particular foods?

These cyclical food cravings can be tied to the increased level of galanin, which appears to work with estrogen to activate the urge for foods high in fat. This rise in galanin accompanied by a decrease in serotonin may contribute to the cravings that about a third of us encounter during premenstrual syndrome (PMS). This does not surprise us, and is one of the reasons why many nutritionists recommend that you eat more complex carbohydrates during this time to increase the serotonin levels and balance out the chemicals in your brain. In fact, a closely related study from the Premenstrual Syndrome Center at the University of Tennessee Health Sciences Center found that women experiencing PMS felt happier and more relaxed within one hour of drinking special high-carbohydrate liquid meals compared to high-protein meals, which did not evoke such feelings.

For sure, these effects of food on mood may vary among people and be stronger in some than in others, but they are very real. We want you to tune in to your body and the signals that it sends you, for it just may be your neurotransmitters talking instead of a growling stomach.

Tip #6: If foods do not help your moodiness, review the depression checklist. If you find moodiness is not affected by your food choices and you feel sad or disinterested much of the time, you may be depressed. Depression is not a character flaw, it is a very treatable medical condition. In fact, depression is seen more often in women than in men, it runs in families, and tends to recur periodically. Stressful events can precipitate or aggravate an episode in someone predisposed to the problem.

Depression Checklist

If you are depressed or sad most of the time or have lost interest in activities that formerly were pleasurable and have four or more of the following symptoms, you need to see your physician or a licensed mental-health professional for evaluation and treatment.

_____   Significant weight loss or gain

_____   Sleep disturbance or increased sleeping

_____   Fatigue or loss of energy nearly every day

_____   Feelings of worthlessness or excessive and inappropriate guilt

_____   Diminished concentration or indecisiveness

_____   Sluggishness or agitation

_____   Thoughts of suicide

STEP #3: WORK WITH YOUR PERSONAL CIRCADIAN RHYTHM

While the foods you eat can play a key role in how you feel each day, your performance and energy level can also be affected by your body's circadian rhythm. Circadian or internal body rhythm, a twenty-five-hour cycle, is kept in sync with the twenty-four-hour day/night cycle through environmental cues such as daylight, darkness, barometric pressure, and humidity (see Chapter 4). The body rhythm is individually synchronized, and thus is the reason why some people identify themselves as early birds while others function better as night owls.

Your body can be thrown out of sync when you travel across time zones (jet lag), rotate on shift work, change the clock for daylight saving time, or when you stay up late and sleep in on weekends. Caffeine and alcohol can also interfere with the sleep-wake cycle of your circadian rhythm. The resulting fatigue, irritability, and shortened attention span can affect performance negatively.

Tip #1: Adjust your work schedule for maximum performance. Psychologists have shown that jobs requiring logic and memory are best tackled in the morning while repetitive tasks are better carried out in the afternoon. But remember that although this tactic may work fine for early birds, night owls may need to adjust their taxing work schedule according to their internal rhythm (clock).

Plan tasks that require alertness and concentration for your peak performance time. If you're an early bird, that's in the morning. If you're a night owl, that will be in the afternoon or evening. During college, both of us were amazed at students who studied late into the night while we set our alarms for 4:00 A.M. to get the most out of our brainpower. Check out what we have defined as the best times for various tasks by looking at both groups.

It's the Best of Times
for Early Birds

Decision making:	Early morning
For your mood:	Morning hours
To eat protein:	Lunch or dinner to improve concentration later in the day
To drink caffeine:	Midafternoon. (Early birds don't need a stimulant in the morning; we're already operating at our peak performance.)
For a Romantic Interlude:	Early morning (While midnight may sound more romantic, both male and female sex hormones peak in the early morning hours. Plus, you're awake to enjoy it!)

For Night Owls

For decision making:	Between 2:00 P.M. and 7:00 P.M.
For your mood:	Evening hours. (The worst time is often early morning hours.)
To eat protein:	Breakfast or early in your day when you need a boost. (Watch eating protein at night, or you may have difficulty sleeping.)
To drink caffeine:	In the morning, if you are forced to get up
For a romantic interlude:	Evening hours because that is your peak mood and energy time

Tip #2: Lower your caffeine intake. There are many ways to lower caffeine intake, but here are some we have found that really work:

- Add up your total consumption in milligrams per day.
- Multiply by 20 percent and decrease intake by that much the first week.
- Continue to decrease by the same amount each week for five weeks until none is consumed.

DECREASING CAFFEINE FORMULA

4 eight-ounce cups of coffee = 560 milligrams
2 twelve-ounce diet colas =   90 milligrams
2 eight-ounce glasses iced tea
or cups of hot tea =   90 mg
Total for day   740 mg
× .20
148 milligrams (to decrease each week)

Week 1: Switch diet colas to caffeine-free.

       Change iced tea to herbal tea.

Week 2: Switch 1 cup of coffee to decaffeinated.

Week 3: Switch 1 additional cup of coffee to decaffeinated.

Week 4: Switch 1 additional cup of coffee to decaffeinated.

Week 5: Switch last cup of coffee to decaffeinated.

DECREASING CAFFEINE WORK SHEET

_____ eight-ounce cups of coffee	= _____	milligrams
_____ twelve-ounce colas	= _____	milligrams
_____ eight-ounce glass(es) iced tea or		
cups of hot tea	= _____	milligrams
Total for day	_____	milligrams
	× __.20	
(Decrease by this amount each week)	_____	milligrams

Tip #3: Use caffeine in moderation after you have decaffeinated. Once you have been without caffeine for several weeks, you can use it judiciously in small amounts for a jolt of energy or alertness. It's the dependence of regular intake that seems to pose the problem for most people. Caffeine addicts will be happy to know that the benefits in terms of alertness and concentration can be achieved at low doses of 20 to 200 milligrams (or one cup of coffee).

Tip #4: Evaluate your anxiety level as you de-stress. Some anxiety is normal and even healthy, because it motivates us to do what we need to do. But there are anxiety disorders that make up the most common mental-health problems. Anxiety disorders include panic attacks, phobias, obsessive-compulsive disorder, and acute or post-traumatic stress disorder, and are very treatable. If you have excessive anxiety or worry occurring more days than not for at least six months and you find it difficult to control the worry, check the following list of symptoms. If you have three or more of these, consult your physician or a licensed mental-health professional for evaluation and treatment.

ANXIETY CHECKLIST

_____ Restlessness or feeling keyed up or on edge

_____ Easily fatigued

_____ Difficulty concentrating or mind going blank

_____ Irritability

_____ Muscle tension

_____ Difficulty sleeping

STEP #4: RESET YOUR CIRCADIAN CLOCK

Whether you are suffering from lack of sleep due to stress or working the night shift, you can use some sleep-enhancing tips to reset your circadian clock.

Tip #1: Control your clock with foods. Here are some ways to use food to help your Circadian cycle work _for_ you.

- Start your day, no matter what time you get up, with foods based on your circadian rhythm. If you are a night owl, you need high-protein foods first (energy boosters), then add the carbohydrate foods (relaxers) as the day progresses. If you are an early bird, save your protein foods for later in the day—lunch and midafternoon—when you need an alertness boost.
- Eat lightly for the several hours before you go to bed.
- Cut off caffeine within four hours of bedtime.
- Avoid alcohol near bedtime.

Tip #2: Adjust your sleeping habits. Some ways you can do this are:

- Try to sleep in one long period, if possible.
- Nap consistently. If you nap, try to take naps at the same time every day.

- Do not try to force yourself to sleep. If you can't go to sleep, do something relaxing until you feel sleepy.
- Make the environment conducive to sleep. Eliminate sounds like phones, keep the room temperature cool, adjust the lighting for optimal darkness, and try earplugs, if necessary.
- Sleep only as much as you need to feel refreshed.
- Wake up at the same time each day, weekday or weekend.
- Have a light snack before you go to sleep to avoid waking up hungry during the night.
- Cut off alcohol and caffeine within four hours of bedtime.

Tip #3: Try exercise and movement to help you sleep. Aerobic exercise is important for health and for sleeping. Get on a regular schedule as outlined in Stress-Less Strategy #3, so you will be physically fit and sleep well. Make sure you spend some time relaxing to help with sleep, too.

What About Smart Drugs?

Smart drugs include several nutrients, herbs, or hormones that proponents say will improve the brain's metabolic pathways and affect our performance. Many different compounds are being used to affect alertness and performance, such as melatonin, DHEA, tyrosine, and gingko. Preliminary reports from individual users appear promising, but we need scientific evidence as to what doses can safely be used, and over what time period their use is safe.

The only way to be sure is to conduct the scientific studies. Watch for more research on these substances in the future.

In the meantime, you can control stress eating today by mastering the EAT Plan. Now that you understand how to reset your circadian clock and use food effectively to enhance or change your mood, it's time to learn how to increase happy hormones in Stress-less Strategy #3: Discover the Magic of Movement.

CHECKLIST FOR STRESS-LESS STRATEGY #2

_____   Take your Personal Food Barometer.

_____   Use food to help your mood.

_____   Work with your personal circadian rhythm.

_____   Reset your circadian clock.

STRESS-LESS STRATEGY #3: DISCOVER THE MAGIC OF MOVEMENT

"I can't believe it, but it's working. After I walk each morning before going to the office, I feel as if a dark cloud has lifted. I see life so much differently." Carmen seemed pleasantly surprised that moving around more could help to eliminate the effects of harmful stress on her body. "Getting out of bed and putting on my sweats before work was the last thing I wanted to do when I'd rather sleep, but I'm handling everything so much better. Even my employees have noticed a difference."

Aren't most of us like Carmen, preferring to sleep later rather than get up and exercise? We'll be the first to admit that it's difficult to give up thirty minutes or more each day to rev up the body, especially when lounging around seems so much more inviting. But we also know that movement is part of an attitude game; that is, if you perceive exercise as a necessary evil, you will find any excuse to keep from doing it. We want you to start now, week three, and begin viewing relaxation, physical activity, and exercise as positive steps you are taking for *you*—not because we are telling you to, but because you want to reap great benefits, including dealing with stress positively.

STEP #1: CHECK YOUR ATTITUDE

You hold the key to week #3. However, before you can fully carry out the steps in this strategy, it is important to make a few adjustments in your attitude.

"Attitude? But I've never liked to exercise," you might admit. Well, if it is any consolation, most of our clients who are quite sedentary find that this is the most painful strategy to adopt in our EAT Plan. We know that you are pressed for time, and when you feel over-committed, it *is* difficult to think of adding still another commitment to your daily To Do list. But the benefits of moving around far outweigh the disadvantages.

TWELVE BENEFITS OF PHYSICAL ACTIVITY AND EXERCISE

1. Increase metabolism to burn more calories
2. Improve the quality of sleep
3. Boost brainpower
4. Fight against aging
5. Reduce body fat
6. Help to protect against cancer
7. Strengthen your bones
8. Boost endorphins, improving mood and helping to relieve depression
9. Cut your risk for diabetes, hypertension, and other diseases
10. Improve cholesterol profile (increases protective HDLs)
11. Enhance your self-image
12. Increase your sexual appetite

But we really don't have to convince you that the benefits of movement are incredible, do we? Starting now, with your regular program of physical activity, you are going to experience everything from an increase in your desire for sexual activity to more energy to less anxiety or all of the above, depending on what your individual needs are.

Remember in Chapter 5 where we talked about how regular participation in some type of aerobic exercise had been reported to reduce symptoms of moderate depression and enhance psychological fitness? Exercise can produce changes in the brain-chemical levels, which can have an effect on the psychological state. A low level of the brain chemicals known as endorphins is associated with depression. During exercise, blood levels of this substance increase and may help to alleviate symptoms of depression. Exercise also slows the release of heart-racing adrenaline into the bloodstream—you will feel better and be healthier when you move around.

> Endorphins or "happy hormones" are produced by the brain in response to exercise and create a state of euphoria or exhilaration.

> Adrenaline, a combination of epinephrine and norepinephrine, is produced by your adrenal glands during the "fight-or-flight" response to stress.

Once you start to view exercise and activity as outlets for you that can be really fun, things will start to look a little different. However, it's up to you to decide to make the time for relaxation, physical activity, and exercise and, even more importantly, to have a new outlook about the way you view them. If your attitude is changing a bit, you have just won half the battle. We promise that the other half will be even more fun.

Now, before you get started with Stress-Less Strategy #3, go ahead and take an inner glimpse with an attitude check. Remember Carmen? We have found that often an attitude like Carmen's can hinder a desire to make lifestyle changes, while a positive attitude can give you the much-needed boost to get started, especially when it comes to making a commitment to exercise and activity.

Use the following Attitude Check to measure your attitude.

ATTITUDE CHECK

1. What is your attitude toward relaxation? Physical activity? Exercise?

2. Do you have negative experiences regarding exercise or activity? If so, what type of attitude adjustment must you make before you can move further with this program?

3. Do you need to unwind before you participate in physical activities or exercise, or do these activities enable you to unwind?

4. Reviewing the relaxation tools listed in Chapter 5, which type of relaxation activity would you enjoy? (Music, aromatherapy, guided imagery, etc.)

5. Do you prefer physical activities (such as gardening, cleaning the house, playing with the kids, or walking the mall) to exercise (such as riding a stationary bike or walking on an electronic treadmill)? Which are your favorites?

6. What do you want to achieve by exercising? Lose weight? Develop or tone muscles? Improve cardiovascular endurance? De-stress? Feel more energetic?

7. How many times a week do you want to work out and/or participate in some physical activity? _____

8. How much time can you spend exercising?

_____

9. Can you do some type of physical activity daily, even if it is just
   taking the stairs at work or parking farther away from the grocery
   store? If so, what?

_____

10. What are the benefits of exercise and activity that are most attrac-
    tive to you?

_____

STEP #2: CHOOSE EXERCISES AND ACTIVITIES THAT WORK FOR YOU

Drawing from the answers above, you can begin to develop a physical activity and exercise program that you will have fun with, particularly if you have made a commitment to view movement in a different light. Keep in mind, however, that no matter what you do, consistency is the key. The more consistent you are, the more these activities will become a part of your daily life, and you can achieve the goals you have set.

To stay with Stress-Less Strategy #3, it is important to choose exercises and activities that you enjoy. Check the following that appeal to you or add your favorites to the list:

Exercise and Activity

____	Badminton	____	Cleaning
____	Baseball	____	Dancing
____	Basketball	____	Gardening
____	Biking	____	Golf
____	Bowling	____	Handball
____	Calisthenics	____	High-impact aerobics

_____ Hiking   _____ Mall walking
_____ Jumping rope   _____ Mowing the lawn
_____ Kick-boxing   _____ Martial arts (karate,
_____ Low-impact aerobics   tae kwon do, etc.)

Exercise and Activity

_____ Playing with children   _____ Strength training
_____ Rollerblading   (weight lifting)
_____ Rollerskating   _____ Swimming
_____ Rowing   _____ Tennis
_____ Running   _____ Vacuuming
_____ Soccer   _____ Volleyball
_____ Softball   _____ Walking
_____ Stair climbing   _____ Washing windows
_____ Stationary cycling   _____ Water exercises

What exercise and activities did you check? Do you like to play golf? Tennis? Ride bikes? Perhaps you find that mall walking while window shopping relaxes you while providing activity. What about yardwork? Mowing the lawn and pulling weeds will keep both you and your home looking great.

Aerobic exercise (meaning "with oxygen") includes such activities as walking, biking, jogging, cross-country skiing, rowing, swimming, playing tennis, or jumping rope. These activities are called aerobic because the body's fuel for performance is produced in the presence of oxygen. When performed regularly, aerobic exercise challenges the heart and lungs, and also will boost your metabolism and control your weight—even during stressful times. In order for you to achieve the maximum benefit, try to perform the exercise at least 20 to 30 minutes, 3 to 5 times a week, at 60 to 80 percent of your maximum heart rate. Working within your target heart-rate range is important, as it prevents pushing your heart at a dangerously high rate of beats per minute, but also makes sure you are exerting enough effort to boost the heart rate into your exercise range.

Anaerobic exercise ("without oxygen") includes strength training and sprint-type activities. These activities are called anerobic because the "fuel" the body uses for performance is manufactured in the absence of oxygen. This form of resistance exercise will enable you to build muscle, raise your metabolism, and tone your body. Examples of strengthening exercises are isometrics and strength training using free weights, resistance machines, or resistance bands.

Whatever it is that you enjoy and will keep doing, we want you to incorporate these favorite exercises and activities into your daily routine. Your goal is for exercise and activity to be pleasurable and not a chore.

STEP #3: SET SMALL AND SIMPLE GOALS

Goals are vital for success in anything we do, and with the EAT Plan, setting goals will help turn your initial enthusiasm into a reality. But without specific goals, you have no way to measure growth. Make sure that the goals you set are specific, and *write these down* so you will visualize the commitment (see page 153). Also make sure that the goals are realistic as you attempt something you can actually achieve. Review these goals frequently and make changes as necessary.

When setting your goals, remember the SAS acronym:

Small and Simple

If you set your goals too high, you will make yourself frustrated and possibly quit sooner because of the difficulty you will have achieving them. Set them small and simple so that once you reach them, you can set new ones. For instance, if you were to start a walking program, set a weekly goal of walking one mile, twice a week. Once you have completed this goal, change it to $1^1/_2$ miles, twice a week. You could also set your goal by time, for instance walking for twenty minutes at first, then progressing to twenty-five minutes, then thirty minutes and so on until you reach the level you wish to achieve.

STEP #4: DO AWAY WITH THE NO PAIN, NO GAIN THEORY

Watch for setting your goals too high, or you might quit exercising altogether, as Shawn did. This middle-age attorney was so enthusiastic about the EAT Plan that he decided to go full force with each of the Stress-Less Strategies. This was great the first three weeks as he learned to be an Active Mood Manager while planning his life to eliminate a lifelong habit of procrastination. But when it came to exercise, this forty-two-year-old man decided that he wasn't going to start small; he was going to go for the gold. In Shawn's case, going for the gold meant running two miles a day the entire first week, although he had not exercised in years.

When we talked with Shawn over the telephone, he was in bed with a moist heating pad on his sore muscles, along with painful shin splints, and he had vowed never to exercise again. We had to remind this overzealous man that by starting one step at a time, his body could adjust to the new physical stress it was receiving. Shawn took the adage "No pain, no gain" to heart and found out the hard way that this adage is not true, especially when you haven't been physically active in some time.

As you make plans to start your exercise program, establish goals that are *reasonable* for your age and physical condition. If you are over the age of thirty-five or have any physical complaints or risk factors, such as diabetes or heart disease, see your doctor before starting any exercise program. With your physician's approval, start your exercise program slowly. The no pain, no gain adage can be dangerous if taken to heart. It is important to spend time warming up prior to exercise by walking or jogging slowly for five to ten minutes in place and then stretching. This warm-up serves to gradually prepare the muscles, heart, and lungs for exercise. It is equally important to cool down gradually so that the heart rate decreases slowly. You also need to stretch to prevent soreness in your muscles.

If you are healthy and relatively fit, work into a regular program of at least 20 to 30 minutes of endurance exercise, 3 to 5 times a week. On alternate days, complement this with a strength-training program, building up to 2 sets of 10 to 15 repetitions using 5- to 15-pound weights or heavier as you are able. Start slowly, listen to your body, and stop exercising when it tells you that it is time to quit.

Suggested SAS Exercise Goals

1. To move around at least twenty to thirty minutes every day with exercise and activity
2. To start slowly, listen to my body, and make this a lifetime commitment
3. To incorporate this time for exercise and activity in my daily To Do list
4. To increase my exercise and activity time each week until I reach my desired goal
5. To listen to my body and back off when it seems too tired or sore

Personal SAS Exercise Goals

1. _____
2. _____
3. _____
4. _____
5. _____

Create an Exercise/Activity Schedule

Once you have thoughtfully established personal exercise goals, we want you to create an exercise and activity schedule suited to your lifestyle. This will vary according to how many days a week you want to move around. Steven, a sedentary computer analyst, found that to move around more, he had to make a point to write in exercise and activity in his daily To Do list. He brought his Day-Timer to show us how he successfully achieved Stress-Less Strategy #3, as follows:

To Do

6:15 A.M.—20-minute walk before work.

7:30 A.M.—Park in back of lot; walk to office building; take stairs to office.

12:00 P.M.—Walk down the stairs to restaurant 4 blocks away/walk back and take the stairs instead of elevator.

6:30 P.M.—Bike-ride while watching news—15 minutes.

Perhaps this does not seem like much activity and exercise, but Steven kept tabs on the amount of time spent, and he averaged almost one hour a day of aerobic exercise—enough to help improve his mood, reduce his mild hypertension (high blood pressure) to a safe range, lower his resting heart rate, and reduce his weight by seven pounds in two months *without reducing calories*. Now that is impressive, isn't it? We think so.

Checking Your Pulse

After your warm up, take your pulse. You can find a pulse by placing your finger (not your thumb) on the artery on the side of your windpipe (your carotid pulse) or on the thumb side of the wrist. Count your pulse rate for fifteen seconds. Multiply this number by four to get your total pulse for one minute. Speed up or slow down your pace depending on your target heart rate range. About 10 minutes into your workout, check your pulse again.

Your target heart-rate range will vary depending on your age. To compute your heart-rate range, subtract your age from 220 and multiply this number by 60 percent. This gives you the low end of your range. Now subtract your age from 220 and multiply this number by 80 percent to get the high end of your range. It is important to keep your heart rate in this zone while exercising.

SAMPLE TARGET HEART RATE RANGE FOR AGE 35
$220 - 35 = 185 \times 60\% = 111$
$220 - 35 = 185 \times 80\% = 148$
Target Heart Rate Range: 111–148

SIX-WEEK ACTIVITY
AND RELAXATION RECORD

WEEK	MONDAY	TUESDAY	WEDNESDAY	THURSDAY	FRIDAY	SATURDAY	SUNDAY
1	Activity	Activity	Activity	Activity	Activity	Activity	Activity
	Time	Time	Time	Time	Time	Time	Time
	Relaxation	Relaxation	Relaxation	Relaxation	Relaxation	Relaxation	Relaxation
	Time	Time	Time	Time	Time	Time	Time
2	Activity	Activity	Activity	Activity	Activity	Activity	Activity
	Time	Time	Time	Time	Time	Time	Time
	Relaxation	Relaxation	Relaxation	Relaxation	Relaxation	Relaxation	Relaxation
	Time	Time	Time	Time	Time	Time	Time
3	Activity	Activity	Activity	Activity	Activity	Activity	Activity
	Time	Time	Time	Time	Time	Time	Time
	Relaxation	Relaxation	Relaxation	Relaxation	Relaxation	Relaxation	Relaxation
	Time	Time	Time	Time	Time	Time	Time
4	Activity	Activity	Activity	Activity	Activity	Activity	Activity
	Time	Time	Time	Time	Time	Time	Time
	Relaxation	Relaxation	Relaxation	Relaxation	Relaxation	Relaxation	Relaxation
	Time	Time	Time	Time	Time	Time	Time
5	Activity	Activity	Activity	Activity	Activity	Activity	Activity
	Time	Time	Time	Time	Time	Time	Time
	Relaxation	Relaxation	Relaxation	Relaxation	Relaxation	Relaxation	Relaxation
	Time	Time	Time	Time	Time	Time	Time
6	Activity	Activity	Activity	Activity	Activity	Activity	Activity
	Time	Time	Time	Time	Time	Time	Time
	Relaxation	Relaxation	Relaxation	Relaxation	Relaxation	Relaxation	Relaxation
	Time	Time	Time	Time	Time	Time	Time

The following chart gives you estimates for the low and high end of your target heart-rate range according to age.

Age	60%	80%	Age	60%	80%
20	120	160	60	96	128
30	114	152	70	90	120
40	108	144	80	84	112
50	102	136	90	78	104

The Benefits of Cross-Training

Cross-training was initially instrumental in helping athletes avoid or reduce injuries from repeating the same movements every day. For those who are not athletes in training, cross-training helps eliminate boredom while continuing to provide the necessary movement for your body.

We encourage clients to vary their routine, especially if they have difficulty staying with an exercise program. For example, you might ride bikes two days a week and walk the mall or swim the other two or three days. Or you might cross-train within the same day as you walk in the morning, then use a rowing machine or stationary bicycle while watching the news after dinner. Choosing different activities and alternating them will reduce the stress you place on the same muscle group and also keep you from getting board.

On alternate days of your aerobic exercise, you may consider some form of weight training or toning exercises. There are many fitness videos available covering all types of exercises from calisthenics and yoga to body sculpting and step aerobics. To find the one that suits you, rent several videos first before making the purchase. With some of these videos, you may need to purchase wrist or ankle weights, rubber bands, or an aerobic step. If videos are not for you, consider a few sessions with a personal trainer or an exercise physiologist at a gym or health club to get you started with the right program.

WATCH EXERCISE BURNOUT

Symptoms of overtraining include an elevated resting heart rate, deteriorating performance, insomnia, and lethargy. For good self-defense, ease off for a while; then when you are ready to increase your performance, do it SAS!

Purchasing Exercise Equipment

Today we have the option of exercising inside or outdoors. If you do not feel safe outside or only have time to work out after dark, you may want to invest in a piece of exercise equipment. If you want to buy a new piece of equipment, shop around. Consider your budget before you investigate your options, for you can spend from $100 to more than $3,000 depending on the type of equipment you purchase.

Consider the following before purchasing exercise equipment:

Check out the warranty for service and parts. This should be at least ninety days, and in some stores you can buy an extended warranty that will carry over for several years.

Check out the construction. Read books or magazines to find out how the model has stood up to use in previous years.

Shop at a reputable store with salespeople who know their equipment. Make sure that they instruct you on the correct way to use it.

Find out if the equipment comes assembled or if you have to do it. Look at the instructions before you purchase the equipment, and decide if it is better to pay to have a service representative do this.

Try it on for size. Don't be embarrassed! Is it comfortable? Does it fit your body? Is it easy to use? Try out the test model for several minutes to see how you feel on it. Compare several models for comfort and fit.

Do you really need those fancy gadgets? Remember, the price is greatly affected by extras.

STEP #4: PRACTICE RELAXATION TECHNIQUES DAILY

Not only are exercise and activity important in this third week in the EAT Plan, we also want to help you learn to create your personal mini-oasis throughout your demanding day with relaxation techniques. We know personally that relaxation techniques such as aromatherapy, breathing exercises, and guided imagery help us to stay calm in a hectic day and also help us to manage stress successfully. While we explained the eight relaxation techniques in Chapter 5, we now want you to select the ones (or all) that seem most helpful and incorporate these in your daily lifestyle. Using the Six-Week Activity and Relaxation Record on page 155, fill in the amount of time you use relaxation techniques each day, trying to reach a goal of at least twenty minutes per day.

Music Therapy

This form of relaxation can be used two ways: actively and passively. You can use music actively to help manage your moods throughout the day and to express your feelings by playing an instrument or through singing. Cathy finds that singing with Paul Simon while driving home from seminars is a great way to relax. In the passive mode, you can use music therapy by listening to recorded music, such as tapes, CDs, or other performed music to de-stress your body. Susan listens to the lively lyrics of Jimmy Buffet to pep herself up before a presentation and then calms down with the jazz of Kenny G or the soothing sounds of the London Symphony after a day of teaching.

For de-stressing, the pace of the music you choose should be slightly slower than your heart rate, or approximately sixty beats a minute. This rhythm encourages your heart rate to slow, and some studies of late have shown that this will also lower blood pressure. Composers such as Vivaldi and Chopin have works that would fit this category, or you might try New Age music, such as "Autumn" by George Winston.

Aromatherapy

Two of the most popular ways to use aromatherapy oils are in the bath or simmering in a pot of water. Some people mist fragrances into a room with a diffuser. You can use aromatherapy to revive on an exhausting day as you enjoy fragrances that make you feel alert and energetic, using lemon, lime, orange, pine, and rosemary. Or you can use aromatherapy to relax, using oils and fragrances that make you feel serene and soothed, such as chamomile, rose, lavender, and orange blossom.

As a general rule, oils are not to be rubbed directly on the skin, unless they are in the form of a lotion or are diluted with a carrier oil or base oil. Keep all oils away from the eyes and never take internally. Remember, oils are strong and more does not mean better. Oils and aromatherapy products are available in major department stores, health-food stores, specialty bath stores, some discount stores, kiosks in the malls, and by mail order.

To use aromatherapy, put a few drops of oil into a pot of boiling water and enjoy the vapors. Add a drop or two to your bath or use a ring that sits on your lightbulb. To use it, you put a few drops of oil into the ring. The bulb, when turned on, heats the oil and sends the fragrance throughout the room. An aromatic diffuser uses a few drops of oil and disperses these droplets in a fine mist throughout the room. Some diffusers are heated by candles, others by electricity. Oils could even be used in a vaporizer or humidifier.

Along the same idea as aromatherapy is hydrotherapy. These are fragranced bath treatments using aromatic soaps and oils that wash away tension and ease anxiety. Many salons, department stores, and drugstores have different lines of hydrotherapy products from shower gels to bath oils to scented lotions, including Caswell Massey, Crabtree & Evelyn, and Victoria's Secret, among others.

You can get your own spa benefit at home with a sea-salt body rub. Purchase a package of sea salt and a sponge or sisal mitt. Once you are in your bath, sprinkle your mitt or sponge with sea salt and gently rub in a circular motion, avoiding any cuts on the body as you know that salt stings. Rinse and apply your favorite aromatic lotion. While you are relaxing, put cucumber slices or cold tea bags on your eyes, helping to reduce puffiness in some cases.

Guided Imagery or Visualization

While imagery is used to trigger the relaxation response, it is different from actually relaxing because it requires different cognitive processes. During relaxation, your thoughts are free flowing and purposefully undirected. Relaxation is designed to promote rest and calm the body as you forget about the stressful events of the day.

To use guided imagery, allow yourself ten to twenty minutes to de-stress while on your mini-vacation. Close your eyes, take a deep breath, and exhale slowly (let the air fill your stomach enough to push it outward). Visualize yourself in peaceful surroundings, such as walking the beach at sunrise. Try to involve your senses as you do this by listening to the sounds of the waves as they wash upon the shore. Hear the birds singing overhead. Feel the warmth of the morning sun and the cool splash of water as the waves crash on your ankles. Push your feet into the cool sugar sand and relish this mini-vacation away from daily stressors.

Yoga or Tai Chi

For centuries, yoga and tai chi have been used by millions who believe these ancient disciplines help to give an inner peace or calmness. Those who practice this find that the rhythmic motions clear the mind, alleviate stress, and improve mood. The various positions in yoga and tai chi also serve to tone the body and help to build muscle strength as you do various exercises, while maneuvering your joints in relaxing range-of-motion movements.

Deep Abdominal Breathing

Diaphragmatic breathing or deep abdominal breathing can help to relax you, even during the moment of stress. Breathing is one of the involuntary activities of the body that we can consciously control. Once put into practice, it can help to decrease the release of stress hormones and slow down your heart rate during stressful moments.

Lie down on the floor or bed, and place your hands on your stomach or abdomen. As you breathe in through your nose, let the air fill your stomach and feel it press against your hands. Slowly exhale through your mouth as you very lightly press your hands against your stomach, letting out all of the air. Repeat this two or three times, and practice this exercise so that when you are facing stress, such as giving a presentation or a meeting with your boss, you can do deep abdominal breathing to ease the tension and calm your anxiety.

Massage

As we discussed in Chapter 5, the benefits of massage include heightened alertness, relief from depression and anxiety, an increase in the number of natural "killer cells" in the immune system, lower levels of the stress hormone cortisol, and reduced difficulty in getting to sleep.

To get started with massage, you need to find a licensed massage therapist (LMT). Check with area wellness centers or ask your physician for a reference. Many full-service hair salons, spas, and exercise facilities have LMTs on staff.

Progressive Muscle Relaxation

Lie down or sit down in a comfortable place with no stimulation in the surroundings. If necessary, take the phone off the hook so you can experience total peace. Take a few deep breaths using the method described under "Deep Abdominal Breathing" (page 161), then, one at a time, concentrate and tense each major muscle group in the body, beginning with the head, neck, and shoulders and going down to the pelvis, legs, and feet. After you have tensed the muscle group, relax it for about thirty seconds and continue on to the next group. Once you practice this technique, you can also do it when faced with a stressful situation.

Laughter Therapy

Winston Churchill said, "It is my belief, you cannot deal with the most serious things in the world unless you understand the most amusing." Don't you agree that a really good belly laugh helps you to relax? Why don't you try it right now? We give you permission to laugh aloud—not just a timid giggle, but a real body-shaking guffaw. For men this may be routine, but women tend to cover their mouths and giggle softly. In fact, women not only don't belly laugh; they're not supposed to have a belly! Think of that great joke your friend told you. Go ahead, put a broad smile on your face and laugh until your body shakes with hilarity for thirty seconds. How did you feel after doing this mind/body exercise? Most people will admit that forcing a smile on their face, even when they are grumpy, helps to alleviate some of the tension in their body and stress in their life.

Look at the following two lists and compare how you feel when reading each word.

Happy Words	Gloomy Words
Cheerful	*Depressed*
Smile	*Frown*
Giggle	*Gloom*
Chuckle	*Sob*
Pleasant	*Cantankerous*
Amiable	*Grouchy*
Lighthearted	*Dull*

LIGHTEN UP THE DARKEST DAY

- Call a friend who is fun to be around and go to a humorous movie together.
- Listen to your favorite comedian.
- Watch cartoons with your children or by yourself.
- Take a step back in time and go to an amusement park with a friend.
- Have a lighthearted weekend and rent several humorous videos.
- Watch humorous sitcoms instead of dramas.
- Turn off the evening news and read the newspaper comics or humorous magazines.

CHECKLIST FOR STRESS-LESS STRATEGY #3

_____ Check your attitude each day.
_____ Choose exercise and activity that work for you.
_____ Mark your calendar and include activity, relaxation, and exercise.
_____ Do away with the "no pain, no gain" theory.
_____ Practice relaxation techniques every day.

STRESS-LESS STRATEGY #4: START PRIORITY PLANNING

Now that you have mastered three stress-less strategies in the EAT Plan, let's move into Week 4 and figure out how to give some order to your harried life. We have experienced that while stress is not going away, it *can* work for you if you have a daily schedule to follow. In Stress-Less Strategy #4, making a list and checking it twice will take on new meaning as you learn to prioritize your life—on paper.

We believe that it is vital to put yourself at the top of your To Do list as you make a weekly schedule of all your commitments and activities, then evaluate your schedule for activities you can say no to. The remaining activities will then be prioritized on your daily To Do list. We have seen that some of our busiest, most productive clients are also the least stressed. Why? Because they learned early on that in order to get it all done, they had to schedule how they spent their time each day.

Opt for Voluntary Simplicity

Voluntary simplicity, a term you are going to hear more and more, is a trend of the nineties. Voluntary simplicity means adopting a more simple lifestyle. It has been referred to by some as "downshifting," where people actually choose to earn less money and purchase fewer things. In other words, people are choosing to get off the fast track with a lifestyle that allows for more free time and a lower stress level. According to a poll commissioned by the Merck Family Fund, 28 percent of a nationwide cross-section of Americans had changed their patterns of consumption by downshifting, opting for more time at home with the family and less income. Many respondents also said that they wanted a more calm, balanced life with less stress. According to the *New York Times*, The Trends Research Institute of Rhineback, New York, has picked up voluntary simplicity as one of its top ten trends for the nineties and the new century. Whether or not this concept is for you, certainly a more balanced, nourishing lifestyle can benefit all of us.

STEP #1: EVALUATE COMMITMENTS AND RESET PRIORITIES

"The problem is not too many commitments," Rachel said. "It is too little time. There is just not enough time to do all I have to do." Do you, like Rachel, find that no matter how you juggle your responsibilities, there is never enough time in the day? Setting priorities and budgeting your time each day is the first step in gaining balance in your life. And having a balanced life can help you deal with life's stressors more effectively.

Before you start reorganizing your life, let's do a reality check. There are only twenty-four hours in each day—so, depending on how much you sleep, you have available to you about sixteen hours of awake time. Following are some guidelines for carrying out your reality check.

List all commitments. Using the form on page 168, make a list of all the commitments you have each week, then check off those that are most essential. Fill this page with your current obligations, including work, family commitments, and community involvement. Be sure to include on this list such important personal needs as exercise, rest, and relaxation. We encourage commitments like spending time with families and loved ones, attention to work, personal renewal, relaxation, and exercise, for these are all vital to achieving balance in your life. When you start adding to your list a host of volunteer commitments, evening meetings, career obligations, or other activities, you could face overload, resulting in additional stress. You need to pick and choose where to draw the line—and no one can draw this line but *you*.

Divide your list into two sections. After you have completed your list of activities and commitments, prioritize these, and divide this list into two sections: A and B. Section A will be those commitments that you cannot change; section B will be those that are more flexible, that you can choose to keep or not.

Schedule your week for peak efficiency. For most of us, staying employed is a major commitment we must keep to put food on the table, but working late into the evening hours or working seven days a week is a commitment we can change. Activity is important to reduce the harmful effects of stress on the body, so add this to the "A" list. We give you permission to stop trying to keep your house so spotless, so put housekeeping on your "B" list, and get it done as you find extra time or delegate jobs to family members.

Be selective about your commitments. After you prioritize your list, cross off those commitments that are not vital to your health or your family's well-being. What changes do you need to make in your list of priorities? Work on what you can change (list "B" or less important tasks), and accept what you can't (list "A" or essential tasks). Just be sure to stay on top of the time spent on all commitments so that your main priorities get done each day.

Prioritize both lists. You can then number the items on list A in order of their priority so you can become more focused and attend to the items that must receive your attention first. Some people find that crossing off each item as they complete it gives them a sense of accomplishment. Divide large tasks that seem overwhelming into smaller parts that can be accomplished in more realistic time slots, and complete one at a time. Also start with item #1 on your A list at the most productive time of the day. Think about when your mind is most clear, and you can focus and really get things done (read pages 82 to 86 on circadian rhythms to see when your alert time of day is).

On Annie's list (shown on page 167), she found that she could cut back on her job hours and drop some volunteer commitments so she would have time out for personal renewal and participation in family activities. We cannot stress enough that taking time out for yourself is vital as you learn how to make stress work for you. Without this downtime, it is virtually impossible to recharge and then reapproach your stressful situations with a renewed spirit.

Set reasonable expectations. As you prioritize your list of commitments, be sure to set reasonable expectations. A constant push for perfection can cause undue stress, which results in hazards to our mental and physical well-being, and researchers are finding that perfectionism may be a key risk factor in burnout. Some of these commitments are bound to be making dents in your schedule and are significant wasters of your valuable time.

Notice how Annie had to choose what was most important in her life as she quit being "all things to all people"? That is a most important step in reducing stress. As we told Annie, realize that you are human, *not perfect*, even though you are pressing on to become something more than you are now. Give yourself permission to lighten up a little and relax so that you can enjoy your life and experience a greater sense of well-being and joy.

PRIORITIZE YOUR LIFE

1. Label "A"—These are the essential commitments you must keep.
2. Label "B"—These are the commitments that are not as important and that you can change.

Annie's Personal Commitment Work Sheet (sample)

1. Get kids off to school
2. Work daily 8:30–3:00
3. Take laundry to cleaners
4. Little League team mother
   (2 hours a day—weekdays/4 hours—Saturday)
5. PTA committee Tuesday nights (3 hours)
6. Volunteer for carnival—Thursday evenings (4 hours)
7. Make costumes for play—10 hours total
8. Telephone committee—3 hours a week
9. Laundry/grocery shopping—daily
10. Time with husband
11. Garage needs painting
12. Garden needs weeding
13. Exercise
14. Kids' homework
15. Make meals for mother
16. Plan family reunion at my house for Thanksgiving
17. Freelance accounting for Ben's business
18. Keep Carol's kids on Monday nights
19. Make curtains for bedroom
20. Relax?!

Annie's Priority Work Sheet (sample)

A

1. Work daily 9:00 A.M.–1:00 P.M.

2. Get kids off to school
3. Time with husband
4. Laundry/grocery shopping
5. Daily exercise program

6. Help with kids' homework
7. Make meals for mother
8. Relax!

B

1. PTA committee Tuesday nights

2. Little League team mother
3. Volunteer for fund-raiser
4. Gardening (exercise!)
5. Chairman of telephone committee

6. Paint garage
7. Keep Carol's kids
8. Make curtains

YOUR PERSONAL COMMITMENT WORK SHEET

(List all commitments here.)

1. _____
2. _____
3. _____
4. _____
5. _____
6. _____
7. _____
8. _____
9. _____
10. _____

11. _____
12. _____
13. _____
14. _____
15. _____
16. _____
17. _____
18. _____
19. _____
20. _____

YOUR PRIORITY WORK SHEET
(Prioritize commitments here.)

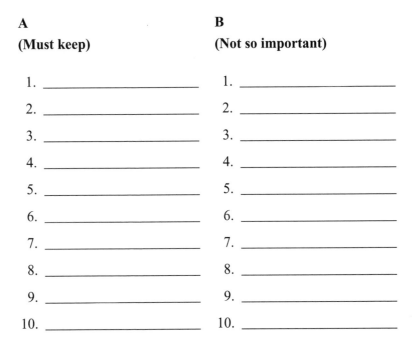

A

(Must keep)

B

(Not so important)

1. _____   1. _____

2. _____   2. _____

3. _____   3. _____

4. _____   4. _____

5. _____   5. _____

6. _____   6. _____

7. _____   7. _____

8. _____   8. _____

9. _____   9. _____

10. _____   10. _____

Lessen your stress. For the commitments (A) that you must keep, identify two ways that you can help lessen the stress caused by each. For example, if you are a parent and must work outside the home, you can lessen the stress of too many responsibilities during evening hours by (1) delegating household chores and (2) cooking quick and easy meals ahead of time. Do the same for those "B" commitments that are more flexible, and write down how you can reduce the stress of these in your life. A sample has been done for you.

Annie's Ways to Reduce Stress

Commitment: Work/family/volunteering.

(1) *Cut back on hours at work.*

(2) *Give up volunteer commitments at night.*

Commitment: Exercise and downtime

(1) *Schedule thirty minutes a day on my daily To Do list.*

(2) *Buy a used treadmill so I can exercise while the kids are at home.*

Commitment: Relax/spend time with husband

(1) *Listen to relaxing music together—without kids around.*

(2) *Go on a long walk after dinner together.*

PERSONAL STRESS REDUCTION WORK SHEET

Commitment: _____

   (1)

   (2)

Commitment: _____

   (1)

   (2)

Commitment: _____

   (1)

   (2)

Commitment: _____

   (1)

   (2)

Commitment: _____

   (1)

   (2)

STEP #2: TREAT YOURSELF LIKE ROYALTY

Now that you are getting a clear picture that in order to reduce the effect of stress on your life you have to learn effective planning, it is time to start treating yourself like royalty.

Here are three nutrition tips to help you be the best you can be each day with plenty of energy so that you can stay alert and be efficient in all you do. We want you to design an eating plan for energy and weight control. We call it eating like royalty, where you will eat like a king, a prince, and a pauper.

BENEFITS OF EATING LIKE ROYALTY	
Less stress	Look great
More energy	Increased productivity
Feel better	Managed weight

Tip #1: Jump-start your day! Eat breakfast within twenty to thirty minutes of when you arise, regardless of the time of day or night that may be. We know that you may not be hungry early in the morning, especially those who must get up before sunrise to meet an early morning commuter train, but to conquer stress on the EAT Plan, it is important to *rise and dine*, eating breakfast within twenty to thirty minutes of when you arise, regardless of the time of day or night that may be.

Yes, Mom was right when she told you that breakfast was the most important meal of the day, but here's why from a stress standpoint. During the time that you are asleep, your body slows down or, more specifically, your metabolism slows down. When you get up and try to shift into gear without food, your body and metabolism remain sluggish. Think of going somewhere in your car and noticing that your gas light is on. You are driving up the interstate ramp and you say to yourself, "I can make it." Minutes later you are out of gas and must pull over to the side of the road and call for help. View your body as your vehicle; without fuel in its gas tank, it doesn't go very far or very

efficiently. When you skip breakfast, it is very difficult for your body
to run like the high-performance machine it is designed to be.

You may be thinking, That's fine for you. You know how to
organize your meals, but I don't have time for breakfast, much less
the energy to fix it. Well, it's now time for the good news of the day.
Breakfast on the Royalty Plan doesn't have to be the traditional eggs-
and-sausage fare. There are many easy and quick foods that work
great to get your motor revved up. Some of Susan's students at the
University of Central Florida ate leftover pizza, and it's amazing how
much more alert they were in class.

When you eat first thing in the morning, your metabolism gets a
jump start, your blood glucose level rises, and your energy level perks
up. If you exercise upon arising, drink a glass of juice or eat a small
piece of fruit first, and have another snack after you finish your workout.

Start with the recipes for Phyto-Fruit Smoothies on pages 130 to
132 as you whip up easy fruit drinks that will give you an extra boost
in the morning. Then add foods from the following list, and eat breakfast like a king:

- Bagels with fat-free or low-fat cream cheese or peanut
  butter or jelly/honey
- Pancakes or waffles with fresh fruit (whole-grain frozen
  ones are available)
- Oatmeal with fresh fruit (instant is fine)
- Leftover pizza (preferably with lower-fat toppings)
- English muffins
- Toast with low-fat cheese
- Cereal with skim milk and fruit
- Banana bran muffins or your favorite whole-grain variety
  (lower in fat)
- Low-fat granola bars
- Don't forget leftovers or sandwiches (who says breakfast
  has to be breakfast foods, anyway?)

Metabolism: the rate at which your body burns calories.

Rev Up Your Metabolism

Remember, the faster your metabolism rate is, the faster you burn calories, which means they are not going to your chin, under your arms, or onto your thighs. Additionally, you will be able to focus on your day and have the energy to meet the demands of it. Okay, you tell us that when you eat breakfast, you are starving by 9:30 A.M? Great! That means you are burning off all of the calories for energy instead of storing them in places where they show. Your body is signaling it is ready for more food, so let's move on to the next stop.

Tip #2: Eat like a king, a prince, and a pauper. That's right. Eat your largest meal at breakfast, a good-sized meal at lunch, and eat less as the day goes on. Think about most Americans. What do we do? You got it. Just the opposite. We skip breakfast except for that jolt of caffeine from coffee or a soda, then eat a pitiful green salad for lunch because we are trying to "diet," and then by two or three in the afternoon we want to know who brought in the M&M's and where they are. By the time we get home, we are ravenous and will eat anything we can get our hands on just to satisfy our hunger regardless of how it tastes, and nutrition is certainly not a priority.

If it is not realistic for you to eat your largest meal in the morning, strive to eat a prince-sized meal in the morning and have a snack mid-morning. This also means eating most of your calories before 5:00 P.M. Our metabolism is the highest the first 12 hours after waking; during that time you burn 75 percent of your day's calories. The problem arises as most of us eat more than two-thirds of our calories after 5:00 P.M. In fact, clients tell us that they resist food all day because they are dieting, then they break the diet during the arsenic hour (around 4:30 P.M.) and eat the rest of the night, resulting in a binge. Then the next day they tell of experiencing the big guilt trip, saying, "I can't believe I ate the whole thing!" How do they cope? They skip breakfast and lunch, and the cycle repeats itself.

Tip #3: Start grazing. Cows do it, sheep do it; we can graze, too.

Here is a rule of thumb for grazing: if you go more than three to four hours between meals, add a snack or graze. Some people refer to them as mini-meals. You are not eating six full meals a day, but five to six small meals (or more). For example, add a midmorning snack

Figure 10.1

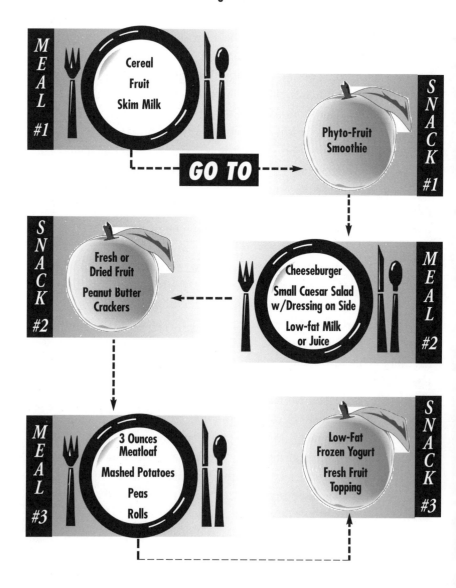

so you are not so ravenous at lunch. Then, instead of eating a cheese-burger, large french fries, and a chocolate shake for lunch, and meat loaf, mashed potatoes with gravy, peas, roll, and pie à la mode for dinner, you will divide your food choices into three grazing meals and snacks as shown.

Remember to add more antioxidants and phytochemicals as you graze for energy. Grazing keeps your blood glucose constant so that you don't become as tired and irritable. You probably know that feeling, too. It is 3:00 P.M. and if no one was looking, you would take a nap. Perhaps your mood also shows that you are tired. Don't think so? Just ask the people around you and see if they think you are a little curt or edgy. Fasting may trigger fat storage, and skipping meals can lead to weight gain. Snacking will help to prevent both. Don't forget the extra bonus: Your metabolism is cranking at a faster rate and burning those calories. A drop in your energy level can also be caused by dehydration, so remember to drink those fluids, especially water.

According to Linda Van Horn, Ph.D., a professor of preventive medicine at Northwestern University Medical School, we should be eating every three to four hours. The advantages of this are important for weight loss, as your body, like your car, will not run out of gaso-line and blood glucose levels remain stable. Providing a steady supply of glucose to the brain helps to prevent negative mood swings and lessens the likelihood of cravings.

The goal with mini-meals is not to eat more food, but to take the amount of food you normally eat and divide it throughout the day more evenly. Van Horn's studies indicated that people eating 1,800 calories in mini-meals versus the same number of calories in only two meals a day lost more weight.

What makes the best snacks to graze on? Some of you will find that your body does great with a carbohydrate snack such as popcorn or a granola bar. Others really need a protein source with their carbo-hydrate in order to keep their blood glucose even and prevent the roller-coaster ride that some people experience when they eat carbo-hydrate alone. Remember that protein foods also help many people to feel more alert, particularly in the afternoon.

Grazers

Veggies with salsa

Phyto-fruit smoothies (see recipes on pages 130 to 132)

Glass of lowfat or skim milk and a pumpkin muffin or banana bread

Granola bar and lowfat yogurt

Small bean burrito

Trail mix

Slice of cheese pizza

String cheese and high-fiber crackers

Popcorn sprinkled with Parmesan cheese

Rice cakes and chocolate lowfat milk

Turkey and lowfat cheese sandwich

More Energy and Weight Loss, Too?

Right now, you might not believe us, but if you incorporate these three tips into your eating habits, you will probably find that you can lose about ten pounds in three to six months without making any other changes at all. Why? Because your body is using calories much more efficiently, rather than being starved all day long and then stuffed with calories that are not burned up but have to be stored in all the places we don't want them.

Janell stared at us as we shared Stress-Less Strategy #4 with her. "I can tell you right now that all I see with this EAT Plan are an escalating scale and thicker thighs," she said doubtfully. If you also think that you will gain weight eating all the time, toss that thought out the window. If your diet has been a dinosaur, remember that it takes a little time to readjust your thinking. Remember the attitude adjustment we talked about?

How Many Calories Do You Need?

Here's an easy way to figure out how many calories your body needs each day:

To estimate your daily calorie needs, start with your desired weight in pounds. Multiply this by 10 if you are a woman and 11 if you are a man. That yields your basal metabolic requirement. Then, decide which of the following best describes your highest level of regular exercise and select the corresponding activity factor:

Sedentary 1.40
Light
(housework, cooking, short stroll) 1.60
Moderate
(brisk swimming or walking) 1.70
Strenuous
(heart-pounding exercise) 1.85

Multiply your metabolic requirement by your activity factor to get your approximate daily calorie budget.

Basal metabolic requirement: the amount of calories essential each day to meet the body's minimum needs.

CALORIES NEEDED PER DAY TO MAINTAIN WEIGHT
WORK SHEET

____ (Body Weight) × ____ (10 [for women] or 11[for men]) = ____ (Basic Metabolic Requirement)

____ (Basic metabolic Requirement) × ____ (Activity Factor) = ____ (Calories Needed to Maintain Weight)

To Lose Weight

To lose weight, take the weight you want to be or your body weight goal (make this a reasonable weight for your height), add a zero to that number, and don't eat fewer than that number of calories per day. This may seem simplistic, but it does prevent people from eating a calorie level below their basal metabolic rate and possibly affecting their metabolism. Perhaps, more importantly, restricting your calories too much will stimulate stress eating, because you are not able to maintain this behavior for a long period of time.

Body Weight $\times$ 10 = Minimum # Calories per Day
If you want to weigh 120, don't eat fewer than 1200 calories.

PERSONAL CALORIE WORK SHEET

____ (Ideal Body Weight Goal) $\times$ 10 = ____ (Minimum # Calories per Day)

Other Helpful Nutrition Nuggets

Lower Fat to Lower Calories. Since fat has twice the caloric value of carbohydrate (9 calories per gram of weight versus 4 calories per gram of weight), it is much easier to lower the fat level and have a significant reduction in calories at the same time. Again the focus is on lifestyle management and looking at your overall nutrition habits, not just at one specific item such as fat. As we mentioned earlier, fat-free is not calorie-free, so even though you may have heard highly promoted diet programs report that you can switch from high-fat foods to fat-free foods, eat these in unlimited amounts, and still lose weight, this is not true. Unlimited calories, including those in fat-free, or high-fat foods, will still cause you to "wiggle when you jiggle," and, again, that's the bottom line.

Some fat may help you lose. For those who religiously follow a very low fat diet, this may interest you as some new comprehensive studies have shed light on the impact of low-fat diets and why you may stay hungry for hours after such a meal. Researchers suggest that the amount of fat in the diet is responsible for regulating total food intake and that when a lower-fat diet is followed, one of the body's natural cues for telling us when we have had enough food is altered, leading us to eat more.

HOW MUCH FAT DO YOU NEED?

Aim for 20 to 30 percent total fat calories in your daily diet. While this is a low-fat diet, there is enough fat to help you feel full after eating.

Use the following formula to calculate your goal in grams of fat on a 20 percent or 30 percent diet, using this method:

- For a 30 percent fat diet, divide your body weight goal (in pounds) by 2.
- For a 20 percent fat diet, divide your body weight goal by 3.

(Example: If your body weight goal is 120 pounds, the 30 percent goal allows 60 grams of fat per day or 120 divided by 2; the 20 percent limit is 40 grams or 120 divided by 3. So this person should aim for somewhere between 40–60 fat grams each day.

YOUR FAT GRAM GOAL:

____ Body Weight goal ÷ 2 = ____ lower Daily Fat Gram goal
____ Body Weight goal 4 3 5 higher Daily Fat Gram goal

Increase the amount of grains, fresh fruits, and vegetables you eat. Most people take in a large percentage of calories each day in refined, processed low-fat or fat-free products, such as cookies and chips. While these may be low fat, remember that what you eat is more important than what you leave out. We want you to focus on eating natural foods—foods high in phytochemicals and antioxidants (see Stress-Less Strategy #1, page 116).

STEP #3: CONTROL YOUR CRAVINGS

All of us are guilty of eating inappropriately when life's stressors seem insurmountable. But you can learn to be in control. Use the following Craving Diary for one week to get in touch with the daily stress you experience and your food response. Analyze what triggers stress eating each day during the week. After you find a correlation between stress and specific cravings, the EAT Plan will help you make simple lifestyle changes so stress eating is lessened.

As you plan your day, you also must plan what you do and don't put into your mouth. Use the following tips to control cravings:

1. Keep a craving diary. Use the diary on page 181 to get started, and the next time you have a craving, jot down the time of day and the circumstances, as well as your mood. Soon you will find a pattern between certain triggers and specific food cravings. For example, if you always want candy after picking up the kids from Scouts or have a jar of honey roasted peanuts hidden in your desk for a quick snack after every sales meeting, write these cravings down. You can learn to deal differently with the situation that triggers your cravings if you know your food reaction.

After realizing from Chapter 2 that she was a sugar craver, especially when she was under stress, Samantha used a diary to get back in control. This helped her to identify her specific cravings and the situations that triggered them. She was able to make some lifestyle changes to cope differently.

Sample Craving Diary—Samantha

Date	Time	Food Craving	Situation Trigger
8/13	9:30	Leftover cherry cheesecake	Kids missed car pool
8/13	1:30	23 vanilla wafers	Brad's tuition bills came
8/14	10:00	Fudge royal ice cream	Washing machine jammed
8/14	3:30	Bridge mix	Kids home from school
8/14	6:30	20 animal crackers	Husband late . . . again
8/15	9:45	2 doughnuts/whole milk	Flat tire on interstate
8/15	3:45	M&M's—$1/2$ bag	Kids home from school
8/16	9:15	Chocolate chip cookies	Saturday—everyone home
8/16	4:00	Ice-cream sundaes with kids	They're driving me crazy!

PERSONAL FOOD CRAVING WORK SHEET
(Write your craving observations here.)

Date	Time	Food Craving	Situation Trigger
――	――	――――――――	――――――――
――	――	――――――――	――――――――
――	――	――――――――	――――――――
――	――	――――――――	――――――――
――	――	――――――――	――――――――
――	――	――――――――	――――――――
――	――	――――――――	――――――――
――	――	――――――――	――――――――
――	――	――――――――	――――――――

Eating frequently works to curb cravings. You will not be hungry or feel deprived so you are less likely to crave foods. Therefore the intake of calories does not get out of hand and add on pounds.

2. Consider your emotions. If you know you can stop at two cookies and feel better, great! But if you have a persistent problem controlling your cravings, you may need to look at other areas of your life besides food. By evaluating your lifestyle and working with a professional therapist, you may uncover unmet needs—comfort, companionship, love, security—somewhere else that are only exhibiting themselves as food desires.

3. Be creative. If you crave crunchy foods like pretzels and chips, see if carrots or chewing gum can relieve tension and relax you. Often you can substitute low-fat, low-calorie food for a high-fat, high-calorie food craving without feeling denied. Try two chocolate graham crackers with a soothing cup of hot herbal tea instead of the grab-and-gulp soda and candy bar you inhale on your way.

4. Give yourself time. Many of our clients describe waiting when they experience a food craving for chocolate candy bars. "Once the craving hits, I make myself wait fifteen minutes to see if it will pass before giving in," Lucy told us. "Many times the craving will pass or I will pop a Hershey's Kiss in my mouth instead and it goes away."

Samantha found that if she ate a healthful breakfast, lunch, and a scheduled snack before the kids got home from school, she wasn't tempted to eat enormous amounts of foods high in fat and sugar. Nibbling or grazing can prevent hunger and appetite from getting the best of you.

5. Give yourself permission to eat. Be sure to allow yourself to eat, eat frequently, and include your favorite foods. After all, this is the **EAT Plan**! While nonstop dieting may be part of your food history, it is a surefire way to leave you more vulnerable to cravings. Remember the Deprivation Theory on page 41, that is, we always want what we can't have.

6. Treat yourself well. Decide what really satisfies you and then schedule it a few times a week in reasonable portions. If you are craving sugar, see if you can first satisfy your urge with a piece of chewing gum or marshmallow, both no-fat foods. But if your craving can only be satisfied with the "real" thing, such as a hot fudge sundae, then work a small portion into your meal plan periodically. It is better to give in to your craving than to try to avoid it, in which case you might end up overindulging.

7. Make happy hormones. As we have stated, regular exercise, even as little as ten minutes a day, can help you gain control over obsessive food cravings. And regular exercise helps to prevent cravings as it boosts endorphins or "happy hormones," enabling you to handle stress and the subsequent stress eating. Our clients report feeling more in control overall when they exercise, and that spills over into food intake and cravings as well (see Stress-Less Strategy #3 for more on the effects of exercise).

CHECKLIST FOR STRESS-LESS STRATEGY #4
_____   Evaluate commitments and reset priorities.
_____   Treat yourself like royalty.
_____   Give in to your cravings periodically to avoid bingeing from denial.

STRESS-LESS STRATEGY #5: STOP PANIC IN THE PANTRY

Now you know what you're supposed to eat to feel great, but it is not always that simple, is it? Especially when you walk in the door after a grueling day at work or carpooling, preparing a recipe is the last thing on your mind. Though you know you should sauté that frozen skinless chicken breast with fresh veggies, something inside nudges you in a different direction, and you end up eating peanut butter on a bunch of Ritz crackers. For those who are single, cooking meals filled with antioxidants and phytonutrients is even more difficult.

William came to see us with this very problem. This thirty-two-year-old CPA had lived alone since he graduated from college. He came for nutritional instruction, asking, "How can I eat right when I don't even know how to cook?" To look at this lean young man, he appeared to be the picture of health, but his concerns were more far reaching.

"My family's history worries me, as my father and his two brothers all had heart attacks in their late forties," he told us. "I'm working on controlling my stress and have started a regular exercise program. However, it is almost impossible for me to eat like I should."

William would pick up high-fat fast food after working late each night, and weekends were not much better as he snacked throughout the day on the leftover pizza or cheese and crackers. His instructions to us were simple: Teach me how to stock my kitchen and to cook in a healthful way without much time or bother.

Those were some pretty basic instructions, and perhaps while reading this, you might admit that you already know how to do both. But for most reading this book, preparing healthy meals while living life in the fast lane is a challenge. Not only is this stress-less strategy important for good health and immune power, it is also the *key* to stopping unwanted weight gain or weight loss from stress eating as you stop panic in the pantry and arrange your kitchen for quick and nutritious meal preparation.

To help make stress work for you, Stress-Less Strategy #1 outlined how to eat to boost good health (by eating foods high in antioxidants and phytonutrients). In Stress-Less Strategy #2, you learned how to eat certain carbohydrates and proteins to calm you down or pump you up as you became an Active Mood Manager. You will now learn how to put all your new knowledge together as we become your Personal Food Trainers and revamp your kitchen to let stress and your busy lifestyle work for you.

The next twenty pages will help give you a top-to-bottom analysis of your cooking style and your kitchen—your pantry, refrigerator, and freezer—and teach you how to prepare healthful meals and snacks in just minutes. As you learned in Stress-Less Strategy #4 (Priority Planning), organization and planning are essential in coping with stress each day. The same planning is necessary for the foods you buy, cook, and eat, too.

STEP #1: START WITH THE EAT PLAN
COOKING STYLE QUIZ

Before we can assess your pantry and direct you to making healthful nutritional choices, it is important to check out your cooking style.

Cooking is seeing a dramatic resurgence as more and more people look to their homes for refuge from the perils of daily life. Sociologists claim that this "cocooning" or shutting away the stressors of the world is becoming more widespread. Perhaps that is one reason why cooking classes have become very popular as we associate home with comfort and consolation. As one of Cathy's clients told her, "Learning to cook is cheaper than psychotherapy and more fun, too."

In actuality, cooking is a splendid way to be with family and friends in a relaxed environment while doing something positive to nourish and replenish your body, mind, and spirit. To many, cooking at home rather than spending money at pricey eateries is part of the voluntary simplicity approach to life we spoke of on page 164.

 Discover your cooking style.

Check out the following cooking styles, and decide which one best describes you:

1. The Batch Cook. This person cooks only once a week, usually on the same day, such as Friday night or Saturday morning. Batch cooks routinely make one large dish of a favorite item such as spaghetti, lasagna, or chicken and rice casserole, then eat this cooked item all week long. Leftovers? Apparently this does not bother the Batch Cook, in fact, each night seems like a holiday as she heats up her portion from the original "batch" and celebrates this time-saving way of meal preparation.

2. The Scratch Cook. This person enjoys cooking and has become a rare breed today as she takes the time daily to cook from scratch, usually for the evening meal. She appreciates the taste and healthfulness of foods prepared from scratch, takes pride in meal preparation and presentation, yet often feels like a dying sort in today's fast-paced world.

3. The Freezer Cook. This busy person is definitely organized as he cooks on the weekend for the next week and up to a month of well-planned meals. The Freezer Cook's menu is varied as he tries a myriad of foods and recipes. Portions are important, and he allocates set amounts in containers, according to family size. He labels the containers and freezes these for upcoming days. Between cooking marathons, the Freezer Cook does just what he intends—eats his stored food as planned.

4. The Hit 'n' Run Cook. Priority planning is definitely not part of the Hit 'n' Run Cook's life. Madison Avenue advertisers love this impulsive person, as he goes to the store almost daily, never plans ahead, and purchases what appears to be quick and easy at the moment. Fresh ingredients? Oh, he'll add one or two, such as throwing in some sautéed onions or sliced green pepper with the prepared pasta sauce or chopping up some low-fat cheese to blend with the boxed macaroni mix. But this person chooses mostly the preprepared deli or freezer items.

5. The "I Hate to Cook" Cook. Sorry, cooking must not be in the genes for this person. Her refrigerator looks like a desert wasteland with only one or two items, such as generic soft drinks and a half-empty jar of olives left over from last year's Thanksgiving dinner. The "I Hate to Cook" Cook always eats away from home, or when she wants to cocoon at home, she picks up take-out food. Her idea of cooking? Open a container of processed food, warm it up in the microwave, and eat it out of the same container.

The Revealing Truth

Although you may be a combination of two or more of these styles, be honest and select the one that most closely represents your cooking type. Regardless of the cooking style you picked, our goal is to help you choose and prepare foods that are loaded with antioxidants, fiber, carbohydrates, and protein so that you can combat stress eating and heal your body from the ravaging effects of past stressors.

Here are some quick and easy suggestions for each cooking style so that you can maximize your nutrition with a minimal amount of stress and time:

The Batch Cook

- Make each item in your recipe count, asking, "Is this a good source of lean protein, carbohydrate, fiber, or antioxidants and phytochemicals?"
- Make sure the recipe contains a yellow/orange/dark green vegetable or fruit. If not, add one or more when serving your meal.
- Always add a veggie salad, fresh fruit, and rolls or pasta to balance out your batch cooking.
- Remember food safety. Some foods keep for a maximum of only three days in the refrigerator, so consider freezing half of the batch and thawing remaining portions midweek.

The Scratch Cook

- Be sure to modify older recipes to use lower-fat items such as low-fat or no-fat cheeses, sour creams, and soups.
- Make sure veggie choices are loaded with antioxidants (see page 119).
- Make sure whole-grain breads are rich in fiber, vitamins, and minerals.
- Add wheat germ, nuts, soy protein, wheat or oat bran, flax seed, or oats to boost nutrition of homemade items.

The Freezer Cook

- Choose items to prepare based on taste and content of antioxidants, phytochemicals, fiber, carbohydrate, and protein.

- Defrost portion in refrigerator the night before it is to be served.
- Complement portion with fresh fruit, veggie, salad, and/or whole-grain rolls.
- Steam fresh veggies or make salad while portion is defrosting in microwave.

The Hit 'n' Run Cook

- Stock up on and cook from "bare necessities" on hand and cut down on trips to the store.
- Buy fresh veggies and fruit to add to ready-prepared items on the shelf.
- Before going to bed, decide on the next two days' menus so that you only pick up fresh items that are needed from the store.
- Keep a running grocery list on the refrigerator or in your calendar and shop from it.

The "I Hate to Cook" Cook

- Use the lists given in this stress-less strategy and keep a few yummy healthful snacks in the fridge and cabinet for those times you don't want to order out.
- Use the tips in Stress-Less Strategy #6 to make the best choices when eating on the run.
- Consider keeping microwavable foods, such as frozen dinners, pizzas, and popcorn.
- Freeze grapes, strawberries, and banana slices for quick and easy snacks.

TIMESAVING TIPS FOR ALL COOKS

- Use couscous, orzo, and other small pastas in the base of main dishes, as these cook quickly.
- Always start boiling the water *before* gathering together the rest of your ingredients.
- When making recipes, pull together all necessary ingredients and utensils before your begin cooking.
- Look for no-boil lasagna noodles to make lasagna dishes a breeze.
- Add steamed frozen vegetables to cooked pasta for a quick dish, season with a dash of olive oil, and add fresh garlic or one of the flavored vinegars.
- Don't forget to make a double batch of some items like spaghetti sauce or lasagna and freeze one for another night.

NO TIME TO COOK AND COMPANY'S COMING TO DINNER

Pick up the following for ready-to-serve nutritious meals:
- Ready-made pizza with veggie toppings
- Ready-made sandwiches
- Soups
- Chili
- Stir-fried veggies
- Rice and beans
- Bean burritos
- Bagels
- Prepared tossed or fruit salads
- Chinese or Thai takeout

- Roasted chicken
- Hummus and tabbouleh
- Frozen fruit is great to thaw and serve over angel food cake, or use as a salad, layer in a parfait, or purée as a sauce.

STEP #2: REVAMP YOUR KITCHEN FOR STRESS-LESS MEAL PREPARATION

Now that you realize where your cooking strengths and weaknesses lie, let's start revamping your kitchen for ease and speed of meal preparation.

Carefully go through the following checklists as you learn what bare necessities to keep on hand for quick fixes as well as a list for the grocery express line, weekly shopping, or even for call-in delivery. The items with an asterisk are high in antioxidants and phytochemicals.

Always stock quick fixes in the pantry, refrigerator, freezer, and produce bin.

QUICK FIXES FOR THE PANTRY

____   Tomatoes and green chilies*

____   Olives*

____   Dried beans*

____   Dried fruits such as apricots, peaches*

____   Sliced water chestnuts

____   Sugar-free applesauce

____   Sugar-free gelatin and puddings

____   Canned fruit*

____ Low-fat or fat-free soups

____ Canned beans of choice: kidney, garbanzo, black*

____ 98-percent fat-free refried beans/vegetarian refried beans*

____ Whole wheat or enriched pasta

____ Instant brown rice

____ Canned tomatoes*

____ Tomato paste and tomato sauce*

____ Light and Tangy V-8 Juice®*

____ Low-fat pasta sauce*

____ 100-percent juice packs*

____ Skimmed evaporated milk

____ UHT (packaged) skim milk

____ 98-percent fat-free vegetable/chicken/beef broth

____ 100-percent fruit preserves

____ Canola, peanut, and olive oil

____ Vegetable oil cooking spray

____ Low-fat cake mixes and frostings, such as angel food

____ Low-fat muffin mixes

____ Low-fat cookies

____ Low-fat granola

____ Popcorn, low-fat microwave popcorn

____ Pretzels

____ Salsa*

____ Flavored vinegars, red/white wine vinegar

____ Raisins*

____ Sugar-free beverages and hot chocolate—caffeine free, if desired

____ Quick oats

____ Instant oatmeal

____ Cereals

____ Wheat germ*

_____ Whole-grain crackers and rice cakes (seasoned mini–rice cakes for snacks)

_____ Peanut butter*

_____ Soy sauce

_____ All-purpose seasoning

_____ Buttermilk powder

_____ Nuts (peanuts, almonds, walnuts)*

_____ Whole-grain pancake mixes

_____ Cornmeal

_____ Flour: whole wheat and enriched white

_____ Bran

_____ Sugar: granulated white and brown

_____ Sugar substitute of choice, if desired

_____ Honey

_____ Baking powder and baking soda

_____ Vanilla extract

_____ Herbs and spices of choice

_____ Catsup

_____ Pickles

_____ Maple syrup

Some of the most flavorful herbs and spices include basil, oregano cinnamon, dill, pepper, red pepper flakes, dry mustard, cilantro, garlic, sage, cayenne pepper.

When you have a choice, pick frozen fruits and vegetables rather than canned because they tend to contain less sodium, have better flavor, and are often individually quick frozen (IQF) at the time of picking to retain flavor.

Dried beans, peas, nuts, and lentils are great substitutes for meat and can provide the needed amino acids for protein. For example, substitute $1^1/_2$ cups of red beans and rice for two ounces of meat and get 14 grams of protein.

Choose cereals that are low in fat and high in fiber (at least five grams per serving).

QUICK FIXES FOR THE REFRIGERATOR

_____ Pre-chopped fruits and vegetables*

_____ Baby carrots*

_____ Skim or 1 percent milk

_____ Low-fat or nonfat yogurt

_____ Shredded part-skim mozzarella cheese

_____ Low-fat deli meats

_____ Low-fat or fat-free mayonnaise

_____ Eggs

_____ Lemon/lime juice*

_____ Mustard, flavored varieties as desired

_____ Low-fat or fat-free salad dressings

_____ Low-fat or fat-free sour cream

_____ Low-fat or fat-free cream cheese

_____   Whipped butter

_____   Reduced-fat margarine

_____   Corn or flour tortillas (whole wheat, if available)

_____   Salad greens*

_____   Fresh vegetables*

_____   Fresh fruits*

_____   Low-fat or nonfat ricotta cheese

_____   Low-fat cottage cheese and cheeses

_____   100-percent juices such as orange, orange-pineapple,
        pineapple-orange-banana*

Spinach and red-leaf and green-leaf lettuce have much greater nutritional value than iceberg lettuce and are the highest in antioxidants and phytochemicals.

Always choose vegetables with good coloring, such as deep green or deep orange/yellow. Some of best choices are broccoli, carrots, tomatoes, red/yellow/green bell peppers, spinach, and kale.

Look for fruits that are deep in color. Great choices include apricots, cantaloupe, strawberries, mango, oranges, pink/red grapefruit (a good source of lycopene, one of the carotenoids), peaches, plums, and nectarines.

100-percent juice means that no sweetener, such as sugar or corn syrup, has been added; it's pure juice.

QUICK FIXES FOR THE FREEZER

_____   100 percent fruit juice concentrate*

_____   Frozen stir-fry vegetables without sauce*

_____   Frozen berries and fruit*

_____   Whole-grain bagels, English muffins

_____   Low-fat whole-grain waffles

_____   Pizza shells, such as Boboli®

_____   Frozen-ready dough, such as Bridgford®

_____   Sausage patties—soy-based*

_____   Low-fat cakes, pies, pastries

_____   Low-fat dinners

_____   Low-fat pizzas*

_____   Low-fat frozen yogurt

_____   Sherbet

QUICK FIXES FOR THE PRODUCE BASKET

_____   Winter squash (acorn or butternut)*

_____   Sweet potatoes*

_____   Garlic*

_____   Yellow and red onions*

_____   Baking potatoes*

QUICK FIX FOR WINTER SQUASH*

Pierce the skin. Microwave whole for 6 to 8 minutes on high. Let stand 5 to 10 minutes. Cut squash in half and discard seeds. Add 1 to 2 tablespoons maple syrup to each half of squash. Serve immediately.

Keep a running grocery list on the refrigerator door or in your calendar, writing down products before you run out. Spend a little time planning your meals each week and help de-stress your cooking style. Setting aside only fifteen to twenty minutes a week to plan meals will not only help you save money as you avoid impulsive purchases, but you will be able to include nutrient-dense foods containing antioxidants and phytochemicals. You can catch up on quick meal-planning almost anywhere you have to wait—on the commuter plane, in a taxi, in the doctor's office or before a board meeting, or even sitting in the car-pool line after school. As you plan, don't forget to check your calendar for the coming week's commitments, then plan meals you and your family will enjoy.

It is helpful to make your grocery list at the same time you plan your weekly menus. For example, you might make yours on Sunday evening for the upcoming week.

Use the lists on pages 189 to 195, along with your additions, to form your one-stop grocery list.

Organize your storage so you can locate items easily.

- Alphabetize herbs and spices to find these quickly.
- Use revolving spice racks.
- Use step ladder shelves so that all items can be seen. If you can't see it, you won't use it.
- Date spices when purchased, as flavors wear out over time; replenish as flavor seems to diminish.

Make your kitchen work for you. As you focus on reducing the stress in your life, make sure your kitchen is stocked with some of the following equipment to make food preparation a breeze:

Blender
Kitchen scales for weighing ingredients
Kitchen scissors

Plastic cutting board

Food processor

Rice cooker/steamer

Wire whisks, spatulas (rubber and metal)

Sharp knives and sharpener

Mixing bowls

Measuring spoons and cups (1 set each for dry and liquid measures)

Colander

Mixer, hand-held

Garlic press

Grater

Microwave

Toaster oven

STEP #3: COOK FASTER WITH LESS FUSS

We are always on the lookout for faster ways to cook healthy meals. Try the following for hassle-free cooking:

• For a dinner that is low in stress and high in nutrition, purchase a roasted chicken from the deli at the grocery store, add a fresh veggie salad (sold either in the bag or at the salad bar), and whole-wheat rolls.

• Jazz up canned soups with chopped vegetables, leftover meats, cooked lentils, low-fat cheeses, and flavorful herbs and spices.

• Place portions of cooked rice and pasta in freezer containers. Cover and freeze until firm. When frozen, take out of containers and put in freezer bags, or keep in containers and stack flat. Use these when you are in a hurry for "instant rice and pasta," as you microwave on high for 1 3/4 to 2 minutes.

• Quickly cook a vegetable medley by chopping fresh cabbage, carrots, onions, and red and green peppers into glass bowl. Other favorite veggies can be added or substituted, if you choose. Add 2 tablespoons water and cover with plastic wrap. Microwave on high for 7 to 8 minutes. Season to taste. Substitute with frozen vegetables on a busy night.

• Add flavor to bland veggies and beans by adding flavored vinegars or oil, broths, wine, tomato juice, or even fruit juice, such as apple, cranberry, or pineapple juice.

• Store mushrooms in a brown paper bag in the refrigerator. This keeps them from spoiling as the bag absorbs moisture, and allows you to use these in your weekly menus without having to shop each day.

• Blend salsa with frozen or canned vegetables to give a healthy zing. Add beans and serve over rice for a quick meal.

• Try salsa, fat-free sour cream or cheese, or chili or spaghetti sauce on a baked potato or baked sweet potato.

STEP #4: USE EASY, LOW-FAT SUBSTITUTIONS

With the many no-fat and low-fat foods available today, it is easy to take favorite recipes and replace high-fat items with these healthier foods.

AMERICA'S TOP TEN FAT SOURCES

- Margarine
- Whole milk
- Shortening
- Mayonnaise and salad dressings
- American cheese
- Ground beef
- Low-fat milk
- Eggs
- Butter
- Vanilla ice cream

 Read your label. How do you know if a product is high or low in fat? Read the label. Package labels include the ingredients, the calories, the fat content, nutrients, the sodium and fiber content, and much more for the consumer's information (see sample label).

Sample Label
Healthy Choice Hearty Chicken Vegetable Soup

Ingredients: Chicken stock, potatoes, carrots, cooked white chicken meat, water, celery, diced tomatoes, potato starch, corn, green beans, enriched macaroni product (wheat flour, egg white solids, niacin, ferrous sulfate, thiamine mononitrate, riboflavin), tomato purée, (water, tomato paste). Contains less than one percent of the following ingredients: peas, chicken flavor (contains water, salt, and flavoring), salt, chicken flavor (contains salt, flavor, cultured whey, egg albumin), sugar, potassium chloride, spice, dehydrated garlic, onion powder, disodium monsinate, disodium guanylate, spice extract, modified food starch, sodium phosphates, soy protein isolate, dehydrated parsley, beta-carotene for color, chicken flavor (contains chicken stock, chicken powder, chicken fat) flavoring.

Nutrition Facts

Serving size: 1 cup (245 g)
Servings: about 2
Calories: 120
Fat Calories: 20

Amount per Serving	% DV*
Total Fat 2 g.	3%
Saturated Fat 0.5 g.	3%
Cholesterol 20 mg.	7%
Sodium 470 mg.	20%
Total Carbohydrate 18 g.	6%
Dietary Fiber 2 g.	8%
Sugars 3 g.	
Protein 7g.	
Vitamin A	90%
Vitamin C	0%
Calcium	2%
Iron	4%

*Percent Daily Values (DV) are based on a 2,000-calorie diet.

High or Low Fat? After reading the label, you can figure out the fat content of a product by using the following formula:

1 gram fat = 9 calories

If the serving has 2 grams of fat, then

$2 \times 9 = 18$ calories from fat

If the total calories for a serving are 100, then:

$18/100 = 18\%$ of calories from fat

Seek Balance Each individual food does not have to be 20–30 percent fat calories or less. Remember, fruits and vegetables have little or no fat while some foods like low-fat cheese may have 50 percent fat calories. The idea is to balance high- and low-fat foods over the course of the day and week.

LABELS CAN BE CONFUSING

- "Low-fat" means that a product has no more than 3 grams of fat per serving.
- "Low in saturated fat" means it has no more than 1 gram of saturated fat per serving.
- "Reduced fat" means the product has at least 25 percent less fat per serving than the traditional item.
- "Light" means the product has half the fat or one third the calories of its regular counterpart.
- "Fat-free" has $1/2$ gram of fat or less per serving.

Choosing Meat and Meat Substitutes

Very Lean Meat and Substitutes List

Poultry: Chicken or turkey (white meat, no skin), Cornish hen (no skin).

Fish: Fresh or frozen cod, flounder, haddock, halibut, trout; tuna, fresh or canned in water.

Shellfish: Clams, crab, lobster, scallops, shrimp, imitation shellfish.

Game: Duck or pheasant (no skin), venison, buffalo, ostrich.

Cheese with 1 gram or less fat per ounce: Nonfat or low-fat cottage cheese, fat-free cheese.

Other: Processed sandwich meats with 1 gram or less fat per ounce, such as deli thin, shaved meats; chipped beef; turkey ham; egg whites; egg substitutes; hot dogs with 1 gram or less fat per ounce; kidney (high in cholesterol); sausage with 1 gram or less fat per ounce.

Dried beans, peas, lentils (cooked).

Lean Meat and Substitutes List

Beef: USDA Select or Choice grades of lean beef trimmed of fat, such as round, sirloin, and flank steak; tenderloin; roast (rib, chuck, rump); steak (T-bone, porterhouse, cubed); ground round.

Pork: Lean pork, such as fresh ham; canned, cured, or boiled ham; Canadian bacon; tenderloin; center loin chop.

Lamb: Roast, chop, leg.

Veal: Lean chop, roast.

Poultry: Chicken, turkey (dark meat, no skin), chicken white meat (with skin), domestic duck or goose (well-drained of fat, no skin).

Fish: Herring (uncreamed or smoked), oysters, salmon (fresh or canned), catfish, sardines (canned), tuna (canned in oil, drained).

Game: Goose (no skin), rabbit.

Cheese: 4.5 % fat cottage cheese, grated Parmesan, cheeses with 3 grams or less fat per ounce.

Other: Hot dogs with 3 grams or less fat per ounce; processed sandwich meat with 3 grams or less fat per ounce, such as turkey pastrami or kielbasa; liver; heart (high in cholesterol).

Medium-Fat Meat and Substitutes List

Beef: Most beef products fall into this category (ground beef, meat loaf, corned beef, short ribs, Prime grades of meat trimmed of fat, such as prime rib).

Pork: Top loin, chop, Boston butt, cutlet.

Lamb: Rib roast, ground.

Veal: Cutlet (ground or cubed, unbreaded).

Poultry: Chicken dark meat (with skin), ground turkey or ground chicken, fried chicken (with skin).

Fish: Any fried-fish product.

Cheese: With 5 grams or less per ounce such as feta, mozzarella, ricotta.

Other: Egg (high in cholesterol, limit to 4 per week), sausage (5 grams or less fat per ounce), soy milk, tempeh, tofu.

High-Fat Meat and Substitutes List

Pork: Spareribs, ground pork, pork sausage.

Cheese: All regular cheeses, such as American, cheddar, Monterey Jack, Swiss.

Other: Processed sandwich meats with 8 grams or less fat per ounce, such as bologna, pimiento loaf, salami; sausage, such as bratwurst, Italian; knockwurst, Polish, smoked; hot dog (turkey or chicken); bacon.

Hot dog (beef, pork, or combination).

Peanut butter (contains unsaturated fat).

Names of cuts of meat with the words *loin* or *round* are low in fat.

 Alter recipes to suit your stress-less eating. Substitute fruits and vegetables high in antioxidants and phytochemicals for those that are lower when possible. Most recipes can easily substitute low-fat items for items high in fat, such as using the following:

- Low-fat cheeses such as ricotta, low-fat sour cream or cream cheese
- Evaporated skimmed milk in place of cream
- Light or fat-free mayonnaise
- Low-fat soups

More fat-reducing tips:

- Replace one-third to one-half of the oil, shortening, margarine, or butter in a recipe with applesauce or prune purée (both are available in most supermarkets).
- Use low-fat buttermilk in dressings.
- Try blending low-fat ricotta cheese with low-fat yogurt, low-fat cottage cheese, or low-fat cream cheese in pie and calzones.
- Use part-skim mozzarella on pizza.
- Try fat-free refried beans on tacos.

Check out popular magazines (such as *Cooking Light*, *Eating Well*, *Veggie Life*) for innovative light and healthy cooking ideas.

Jazz up flavors with herbs and spices as you reduce fat in recipes.

- Instead of fat, try garlic, herbs, and spices.
- Use salsas, flavored mustards, flavored vinegars, broths, wine, fruit juices, or chutneys. Keep several on hand in the pantry.

VINEGAR: LOW IN FAT BUT HIGH IN FLAVOR

Drizzle a mixture of vinegar, dill, and Dijon mustard onto fish fillets.

Add balsamic vinegar to fresh strawberries and other fruit.

Sprinkle vinegar with herbs such as tarragon over vegetables and salads.

Splash vinegar with ginger into your stir-fry.

CHECKLIST FOR STRESS-LESS STRATEGY #5

_____ Start with the **EAT Plan** cooking-style quiz.

_____ Revamp your kitchen for stress-less meal preparation.

_____ Cook faster with less fuss.

_____ Use easy, low-fat substitutions.

STRESS-LESS STRATEGY #6: HIT THE ROAD RUNNING

If you have carefully fcllowed the steps in Stress-Less Strategies #1 through #5, for the last five weeks, you've almost mastered the EAT Plan. By this time, you should be feeling the positive benefit of letting the stress in your life work for you as you implement the Energy Action Team into your daily routine and experience a greater sense of calmness and control, more energy, and even improved weight management.

We know you are anxious to learn the rest of the EAT Plan, so let's go. It's week six and the final stress-less strategy is for those of us like Kim, who complained about always being on the road. "When I looked for a new car last year, I tried to find one with a refrigerator because I seem to live in my car," Kim said. "If it isn't carting supplies for my job as a pharmaceutical representative, it's carting my three teens and their friends to after-school activities. The problem is that I haven't figured out how to live in the car and eat right, too."

Whether you are a busy mom who clocks in several hours a day of driving for car pools or a career person who must travel for a living, the steps in this chapter will allow you to continue implementing the EAT Plan as you plan your meals for healthful eating while on the road.

Move Over, Ozzie and Harriet

Americans have been called many things in the past decade, but one thing they aren't is "Ozzie and Harriet." We don't mean that being at home with family is unimportant, for we both agree that these intimate times give all of us stability and roots. But the reality of life is that few of us ever eat an entirely home-cooked meal in our own abode. Even if you are a stay-at-home parent, you know how difficult it is to prepare a well-balanced meal filled with nutritious fruits and vegetables when family members have commitments like work, community meetings, and school activities. Most of our clients who have difficulty balancing eating on the road and healthful nutrition tell us that a common saying at home is, "I'll grab something while I'm out."

So if we aren't eating at home, where *are* we eating? As we discussed in Chapter 3, Americans are certainly getting their nourishment somewhere, as studies show that as a nation we are fatter than ever. A revealing study done by *USA Today* on Road Warriors (people who fly more than 100,000 miles a year or stay in hotels more than 100 nights a year) found that 48 percent of the 1,136 people who responded said what we know to be true: They had gained weight in the past year because of their travel diet. Of those, 65 percent gained more than 6 pounds, and 20 percent put on more than 10 pounds, with men gaining more weight than women.

Eating on the Road Adds Extra Pounds

What is it about being on the road or travel that adds these extra pounds? We asked this question to clients, and here are some of their responses:

- Traveling on business makes me feel lonely, so I eat more.
- I don't exercise when I travel and tend to snack all night.
- When I spend long hours carpooling kids, I bring foods to eat and pass the time.
- I make the wrong food choices when I'm eating with business associates.
- I eat too many rich desserts, especially if I eat with other people.
- I eat heavy dinners late at night after stressful workdays.
- When I eat at fast-food restaurants, I usually order the special because I'm in a hurry. It's usually the double hamburger and large fries.
- I eat dinner with clients or business associates, then get bored in my room so I order room service for dessert.

There is no doubt that eating on the road is a major concern for most of us. Whether we frequent fast-food, take-out, or specialty restaurants and eat in airports, train stations, or the car, in order to get a handle on stress eating, we must become *disciplined diners*.

Rather than a nation of Ozzie and Harriets, some have labeled Americans in the nineties "Dashboard Diners." According to a *University of California at Berkeley Wellness Letter*, in 1993 Americans spent 46 percent of their food expenditures on restaurant meals and food eaten away from home. This was an increase from 39 percent in 1980 and 34 percent in 1970, and there's ample evidence that the trend is continuing. Predictions are that soon over *half* of our meals will be eaten away from home.

Is this trend a healthy one? From the standpoint of nutrition, probably not. At the same time that the number of meals eaten away from home has increased, so has obesity. But, as veteran travelers, we know that you *can* live on the road and still control stress eating. Just like the steps in the previous stress-less strategies, it will take some knowledge, along with careful planning.

EATING IN GROUPS

Eating with more people expands not only your party, but your waistline, too! Eat with one companion and eat 28 percent more; eat with a group of six or more and eat 76 percent more.

Benefits of Dashboard Dining

Many of our clients complain and say if they could only eat at home, everything would be fine. We agree. Often it seems better to eat at home because at least you know what ingredients are going into the food you eat. However, we also believe that there are some advantages to restaurant eating: (1.) You don't have the opportunity for second or third helpings that you have at home, even though portion sizes may be large; and (2.) food is not readily available twenty-four hours a day, as it is at home.

In some ways, we have found that eating out is an easier way to control amounts you eat on the road. Let's review how you can implement this control as you eat on the go.

STEP #1: REMEMBER YOUR EAT PLAN PRIORITIES

As you rethink dining out, it is important to remember your **EAT Plan** priorities.

Tip #1: Choose foods high in antioxidants and phytochemicals like fruits, vegetables, and grains.

Tip #2: Choose carbohydrate foods such as breads, cereals, and pastas for their calming effect.

Tip #3: Choose protein foods like lean meats, cheeses, yogurt, or milk when you need a boost.

Tip #4: Remember to eat like royalty and graze.

STEP #2: DEVELOP DINING DISCIPLINE

Philip told of having no discipline when he ate out each night. As a general manager for a large car-leasing corporation, Philip had to travel several states during the week with a different destination each day. "Do you know how lonely it is to eat by yourself day after day?" he said. "I've really tried to do the dry toast, poached egg, and orange juice breakfast, but if something is on the menu like chocolate-chip pancakes or crispy home fries, I immediately order these because they make me smile."

Perhaps these comfort foods brought a smile to Philip's face for the moment, but it was only temporary. When he came for assistance in losing weight from stress eating, he was topping the scales at 240 pounds. Believe us, when we met Philip, he was not smiling.

We know how tempting it is to try the specials in restaurants, and once in a while it is fun to splurge on something as sinfully delicious as chocolate-chip pancakes. But if you eat on the road frequently, it is important to develop dining discipline or, like Philip, you will be wishing you had.

It is also difficult to have dining discipline when you are spending someone else's money. Whitney, a recent college graduate, told of gaining thirteen pounds in six months after her new job as a sales representative for a well-known computer manufacturer. "I've never had a weight problem," she admitted, "so when they gave me the company credit card and said use this for your meals, I was thrilled. After eating college-dorm food for four years, I certainly took advantage of this. I ate rich cheese omelettes for breakfast, pasta with meat sauces for lunch, then the finest lobster dipped in butter for dinner. Why not? I felt like someone's guest."

As Whitney learned the hard way, you can and must become your own "nutritionist" as you begin to analyze the menu when dining out. We want you to start seeing the menu as a list of ingredients you can rearrange rather than individual set items. For example, if you see spinach as a part of an entrée like veal florentine, they can probably do steamed spinach as a side dish. Perhaps you see steamed carrots and broccoli, but it only comes with the fried chicken dinner. Ask for this vegetable medley as a side dish—without butter. Remember: Hold the mayo and the extra cheese; add lettuce, tomato, and onion, please. It does not hurt to ask, and most eateries are delighted to please their patrons.

When you search your menu for meal choices, look first for those antioxidant sources (remember Stress-Less Strategy #1). Build your meals and snacks around those immune-boosting fruits, vegetables, and grains.

Tip #1: Set priorities as you make food choices.

Dining-Out Appetizers

- Look for vegetable soups.
- Eat pastas with tomato sauces.
- Choose grilled mushrooms or other vegetables.
- Ask for bread to be brought early in the meal. Skip the butter.

Salads

- Focus on romaine or spinach (high in antioxidants).
- Choose dressing on the side, so you can control the amount.
- Try tabbouleh, chopped vegetables, or fresh fruit.

Entrées

- Look for vegetarian choices like pasta with vegetable sauce.
- Choose Chinese vegetables and rice.
- Ask for lean meats like chicken, fish, pork tenderloin, or filet mignon.
- Make sure you get a starch, like potato or rice, instead of french fries. (Eat the starch first if you want to limit calories or fat. Most of our fat comes from meat items.)

Dessert

- If you are with a group, order one or two desserts and share.
- Carry a favorite bite-sized sweet with you to eat afterward on the go. (Some lower-fat bite-sized chocolate treats are Milky Way or 3 Musketeers, but any of the miniatures will do.)

What About Fast Food?

Even with all the warnings about fat content in fast foods, people are eating out in record numbers. Latest statistics show that the average American family eats out four times a week. For convenience's sake, after a busy day at the office or at home, or just because you simply enjoy eating out, it is important to know how to choose a healthful meal that will not put on unwanted pounds. And for most of us, we need to think fast—food, that is. It isn't easy, but using the same priorities you learned for dining out as a guideline, you can analyze the menu to make the best choices.

Breakfast

- Look for a scrambled egg and a low-fat muffin.
- Choose a toasted English muffin.

- Try cereal with skim milk.
- Opt for an egg-and-cheese sandwich on a toasted English muffin rather than the biscuit or croissant breakfast sandwiches, which are higher in fat.

Lunch/Dinner

- Go for the plain hamburger in the smallest size.
- Order grilled chicken sandwiches with no "special" sauces.
- Add condiments yourself.
- Ask for "light" mayonnaise.
- Salads are a good choice, but you may find you're too hungry in the afternoon if that's all you have.
- Add a salad to the sandwich meal, and you're less likely to overeat later in the day.
- Look for chili or a baked potato topped with chili for a filling meal.
- Try the chicken burritos or tacos in soft tortillas.
- Ask for a veggie sub, turkey, or ham with mustard.
- Choose pretzels rather than chips to accompany your meal.

Snacks

- Look for the low-fat or nonfat yogurt shakes or cones.
- Ask for animal crackers as low-fat cookie snacks.

STEP #3: PLAN AHEAD FOR HEALTHY SNACKING

For the millions who travel each day, nutritional eating habits are usually left behind. Too often, it just seems like too much trouble to stay on a healthy schedule or even to find foods that are healthful.

The timing of the meals when you are on the road is important, too. Most of us prefer to have the largest meal in the evening; after all, that's usually when we settle into our destination so it makes sense to relax with a fine meal. But this pattern can also sabotage weight control, especially when you are trying to eat like royalty. Remember eating like a king, prince, and pauper along with grazing? In an experiment at the University of Minnesota's Chronobiology Laboratory, researchers fed subjects a 2,000-calorie breakfast—then nothing else all day—for one week. They all lost weight! When the same meal was eaten at dinnertime, the subjects either gained weight or remained the same.

So the question is, How do you cope with busy days on the road that require you to eat out? You plan ahead. We explained how to become your own menu analyzer and choose healthful meals. Now you need to go one step further. Remember the expression "Don't leave home without it"? Well, we want you to realize the importance of this statement—and we're not talking about credit cards. We are talking about bringing healthful snacks and mini-meals with you—in the car, on the plane, or wherever you go. Stuff your purse, pack your briefcase, or even grab that brown bag, if needed, filled with low-fat, healthful snacks to avoid bingeing on soda pop and chips when hunger pangs strike.

Tip #1: Take healthy snack alternatives with you to avoid snacking from vending machines or making convenience-store grabs. Keep the following choices on hand and put these where you will conveniently pick them up as you leave the house. Or keep several in your briefcase or in the glove compartment of your car as your "emergency snack supply."

- Low-fat or fat-free granola bars
- Peanut butter crackers
- Animal crackers
- Vanilla wafers
- Dried fruit, such as raisins or apricots
- Pretzels
- Bread sticks
- Graham crackers

- Ginger snaps
- Rice or popcorn cakes
- Canned 100-percent juice like orange, grapefruit, tomato, or vegetable
- Bottled water

BROWN-BAG BUDDIES

1 cup raisins, dates, or other dried fruit
1 cup pretzels
1 cup reduced-fat cheese crackers (such as Snackwell's)
1 cup dry-roasted unsalted peanuts, walnuts, or almonds
$1/2$ cup M&M's candies (occasionally for an added treat)
Mix together, divide into $1/2$ cup portions, and keep these with you for emergencies. If you don't portion out the mix, you may find that you munch the entire bag at one time!

Tip #2: Pre-order meals on airline flights. If you are flying out of town, the best option is to call the airline a few days in advance and order a special meal. We have found the food to be fresher, and you're more likely to get something you want. We always order the vegetarian meals in advance but the low-fat or fruit plates work well, too. If, as is true most of the time today, there is no meal served, choose pretzels to calm down or peanuts for staying power. Beverages are varied. We don't recommend drinking alcohol on a plane, for it dehydrates the body. Sticking to antioxidant juices, such as orange, tomato or grapefruit, works best. Bring bottled water or select carbonated water with lemon or lime, if you are unsure as to whether juices will be served.

Tip #3: Make healthy choices at airports. Recently the Physicians' Committee for Responsible Medicine did a survey of the nineteen leading airports for travel. They put together a Top Ten list for healthy choices.

Top Ten Airports for Healthy Dining

1. Los Angeles
2. Pittsburgh
3. Vancouver
4. Seattle
5. Albuquerque
6. Chicago O'Hare
7. Boston
8. Salt Lake City
9. New York (La Guardia)
10. San Francisco

If you're stuck in the terminal with a long wait, choose from the following selections that are almost always available:

- Bagel
- Hot pretzel
- Low-fat or no-fat frozen yogurt
- Vegetarian pizza
- Fruit

There will always be some situations that are beyond your control, and even with the best intentions, you will sometimes eat less than ideally, such as that plump chili dog you grabbed as you ran to the gate for boarding. Don't get stressed out over this! Remember, it's only one meal or snack. The main issue with the EAT Plan is how you eat every day, not what you have for one meal or snack out of one day. We believe that travel is and should be an adventure. Move on and think of all the opportunities you have down the road to meet your eating goals.

STEP #4: REDUCE THE STRESS OF TRAVEL

Travel can be exhilarating, or it can be very stressful, especially when you are not in control of your destiny. Oftentimes, the airlines or other carriers can really ruin your plans, canceling flights, changing seat assignments, or making you wait out lengthy delays because of weather or maintenance. Some of this is unavoidable but some potential problems can be minimized. For those who find that traveling adds to their stress load, you can reduce the effects of long hours spent on boats, planes, and trains by using the following tips:

Tip #1: Avoid booking the last flight out to your destination. That way you always have a backup plan. If it's not too far, you can rent a car and get to where you are going. Or, in some cases, you can relax and look upon your trip as an adventure. We ran into a couple recently who had been on a cruise as part of their workweek and were heading home. All of the flights to their destination were overbooked during the day, so they volunteered six times to give up their seats. All in all, they accumulated over $2,000 in travel vouchers in one day, then got home early the next morning!

Tip #2: Get a jump on jet lag. Gradually match your waking and resting hours to your travel schedule and the location of your eventual destination. This may take a few days prior to the trip. For example, if you are going to Paris, and you normally go to bed at 11:00 P.M. and awaken at 7:00 A.M., train yourself to go to bed earlier each night before the trip so you body clock matches your new destination.

Change your watch to the new time as soon as you board the plane or train. Then, before and during the flight, drink fluids continuously. Water and fruit juices are the beverages of choice.

Be sure you begin discovering your new destination the next morning, even if you feel a bit tired. Getting plenty of sunshine will help to set your biological clock and get you back on a normal sleep track.

Remember to eat like royalty as a king, prince, and pauper, and to graze. This will help to boost your energy level before you bottom out.

Tip #3: Consider using melatonin. Melatonin, a hormone available over the counter in drugstores or health-food stores, has been promoted as everything from a sleep aid to an anti-aging and cancer prevention remedy. Even though this hormone is not regulated by the Food and Drug Administration, it has been recommended by some researchers as a way to counter the effects of jet lag. Though the National Institute of Health is sponsoring $50 million worth of research on melatonin at this time, many of these claims will take years to sort out with scientific studies, but some aspects appear promising.

Melatonin taken an hour before bedtime has been shown to induce sleep more quickly and sleep continues longer than with a placebo. For jet lag, the recommendation is to take it at your destination's bedtime to reset your body clock. Though melatonin appears to be nontoxic, taking too much or at the wrong time could make you sleepy when you need to be awake.

At this writing there is very little evidence as to the long-term effects of melatonin or even the doses recommended. If you want to try melatonin, the best idea is to use as low a dose as possible (1 milligram) while you get a sense of what your reaction will be. Sound like an experiment? At this stage, it is. Side effects may include grogginess upon awakening, depression with those who are susceptible, and nightmares for some.

Tip #4: Continue to exercise. While you may not have your usual gym or the neighborhood running route, it is possible to exercise away from home. Cathy has found that carrying her briefcase and seminar materials through several airports during a travel day is quite a workout. Susan uses exercise bands (such as Dyna Bands) that are three feet long and five inches wide as a substitute for weights, while giving a terrific strength-training workout. Exercise bands fold into the suitcase, take up little space, and can be used in the most compact hotel room with no other equipment needed. You can get aerobic exercise running to make a plane, and strength training by lifting heavy boxes or briefcases. You might enjoy bringing your own exercise video, and always tuck those walking shoes in the suitcase in case you want to climb stairs at the hotel—another way of aerobicizing.

Many hotels have indoor pools, so swimming is a good exercise option. If you're not used to swimming for exercise, it will use different muscle groups and have a cross-training effect. If you are in a hotel with a gym, you can use the treadmills or other equipment as you would at home, or try walking the hallways if it is a large hotel.

Be sure to take your portable audio cassette player when you travel so you can use the music relaxation techniques discussed in Stress-Less Strategy #3. Make relaxation exercises like deep breathing or guided imagery part of your travel routine, on the plane or in the hotel room after a stressful meeting. Take time to pamper yourself with a bubble bath and herbal tea, and if you feel stressed, consider ordering room service for a leisurely dinner upon arrival at your destination.

Tip #5: Pace yourself. While at your destination, try to plan your schedule so that you don't do everything in one day. If you are on a business trip, this is often difficult, especially if you have meetings early the next morning. But to avoid the stress that travel can bring, include plenty of rest in your schedule so that you are able to enjoy your time away. Remember the importance of sleep in de-stressing the body.

Tip #6: Take periodic breaks when on the road. If you choose to drive to your destination, make sure you take periodic breaks, not just for food and facilities but to exercise and relax. Get out of the car, even if only for ten or fifteen minutes, and walk around the area. (We don't suggest this at night or in deserted areas for safety reasons.) You may arrive a few minutes later, but you will feel more refreshed as you go.

CHECKLIST FOR STRESS-LESS STRATEGY #6
_____ Remember your EAT Plan priorities.
_____ Develop dining discipline.
_____ Plan ahead for healthy snacks.
_____ Reduce the stress of travel.

KILL FOR A COOKIE
NO MORE!

Congratulations! We hope you now kill for a cookie no more. The EAT Plan's lifestyle changes, which you have made in the past six weeks, are not meant to be a stop-gap or temporary fix-it. Rather, the EAT Plan is intended to become a part of your daily life for years to come. Following the EAT Plan is a process, not an end in itself. Changing behaviors over time that you may have followed since early childhood takes continual commitment.

As we come to the conclusion of *I'd Kill for a Cookie*, we'd like to share with you some exciting success stories excerpted from letters our clients have sent to us about the EAT Plan and how it has helped to change their lives:

Dear Cathy and Susan,

You know the struggles I was up against before starting the EAT Plan two years ago. Not only was I in the middle of a divorce, but it seemed like the demands of my career as an attorney were overbearing. The EAT Plan helped get me through. Stress-Less Strategy #3 motivated me to start taking responsibility for myself, and I began to exercise each day—something I had not done in twelve years. Slowly I began to feel alive again, and the eleven pounds I had gained from stress eating dropped quickly. As one who ate nothing but coffee and sweets all day, changing my diet to include nine fruits and vegetables was not easy! But, now, two years later, my doctor says I am healthier than I've been in a long time. I have not had a cold in months, which is rare for me.

The EAT Plan truly helped me when I was at an all-time low.

Regards,

Carole (age 34)

Dear Cathy and Susan,

Thought you'd want to know that your EAT Plan helped me to lose twenty-four pounds in six months. Not only did the weight come off by eating more fruits and vegetables and exercising for forty minutes each day, but my blood pressure is lower and I feel alert and in control. Whenever I begin to feel tense, I have learned to take time out to do deep breathing and the guided imagery you taught in Stress-Less Strategy #3. It really works! I can feel my heart rate and breathing slow down. Also, learning how to cook helped me to quit the fast-food track I was on. I'm now a master at cooking quick veggie pastas after work, and my creative fruit salads are the talk of the office.

Your friend,

Paul (age 42)

Dear Cathy and Susan,

I must confess that when I attended your seminar, I did not think that your advice would change my life forever. Before I walked through the door, I lived on fast and easy junk food—for breakfast, lunch, and dinner. As a single career woman, I saw no real need to take care of myself, and I have been healthy. But all of these new studies on disease prevention with antioxidants and phytochemicals really spoke to me, especially as my mother was diagnosed with breast cancer at my age (twenty-two years ago).

I am now eating nine to ten fruits and vegetables per day, and it's not that difficult at all. I'm exercising even when I don't feel like it, my weight is controlled, and my skin looks healthier. When I do eat out, I've learned how to "pick and choose" my meal, rather than just take what the specials are at fast-food restaurants.

The EAT Plan is something that will stay with me for a lifetime, and it looks as if that will be for a long time!

Special thanks,

Carmen (age 58)

Dear Cathy and Susan,

Well, it's been almost eighteen months since I started the EAT Plan, and each day is easier. My anxiety levels are lower, and life does not seem so complicated, especially since I learned how to get in charge of my priorities and quit overcommitting my life. My three children are learning about healthful eating, and they compete with each other to see who can reach the magic number nine with fruits and vegetables each day.

Keep up the good work as you share the EAT Plan with others.

Sincerely,

Wanda (age 42)

Dear Cathy and Susan,

Perhaps the EAT Plan kept me from giving up my career. Remember how stressed out I was when I met with you last year?

Well, you'll be glad to know that since that time, life has been good. I left your office wondering if I could ever get in control of my career and family responsibilities, and after some soul-searching and working through my priorities, I am now in control. Also, eating by your Royalty Plan, with a large breakfast and smaller dinner, has helped me to gain control of my weight. I look better and feel great, too.

Thanks!

Matthew (age 37)

Dear Cathy and Susan,

You must have designed the EAT Plan specifically for me. I was a perfectionist who could not handle life if anything was out of place. Then the twins arrived—five weeks early! My perfect life was definitely out of control, and I coped with this stress by not eating at all. By the time I saw you, the twins were three months old and had gained thirteen pounds. I was almost that much underweight and looked terrible.

The EAT Plan set me straight. I began to organize my life, including my kitchen for healthier cooking, and started some relaxation techniques. My favorite is listening to Chopin while the twins sleep—it calms us all down. I'm now back up to a normal weight, and people think I look younger than ever.

Thank you. You helped save my life.

Elizabeth (age 29)

THE EAT PLAN PROMISES RESULTS

We hope that by now you have had a chance to see results from your newly gained insights into conquering stress eating and the resulting changes in lifestyle that you have made. If you have mastered the six stress-less strategies in our EAT Plan, you should be feeling more energetic as well as calmer as you now cope with your daily stressors in a reasonable manner.

As you close this book and continue to use the stress-less strategies each day, it is our hope that stress eating will now be part of your past and a new passion for living will be yours!

ADDENDUM

SHARE YOUR PERSONAL STORY

We'd like to hear from you. Has the EAT Plan helped you in a special way that you'd like to share with others? Perhaps you are now controlling a once out-of-control weight problem, or you are able to do the things that are important in your life without overcommitting yourself to everyone. Which stress-less strategy was the most helpful in reducing your anxiety and tension levels? Do you have a dinosaur diet story to tell?

Your letters can help us as we share the EAT Plan with those around the country.

Write to us at:

5415 Lake Howell Road, # 246, Winter Park, FL 32792.

SEMINARS AND WORKSHOPS

Drs. Cathy Christie and Susan Mitchell do regular workshops on *I'd Kill for a Cookie* and other nutrition topics. If you are interested in scheduling a workshop for your group, write to them at 5415 Lake Howell Road, #246, Winter Park, FL 32792 or E-mail them at Drchristie@aol.com. or Drsmitch@aol.com or http://www.florida-speakers.com

REFERENCES AND
SUPPORTING RESEARCH

Ader, Robert, et al. "Psychoneuroimmunology: Interactions between the Nervous System and the Immune System." *The Lancet.* Vol. 345 (January 1995) 99–103.

Aldana, S. G., and L. J. Silvester. "The Relationships of Physical Activity and Perceived Stress." *Health Values.* Vol. 13 (September/ October 1989) 34–37.

Akabyashi, A., et. al. "Diurnal Rhythm of Galanin-Like Immunoreactivity in the Paraventricular and Suprachiasmatic Nuclei and Other Hypothalamic Areas." *Peptides.* Vol. 15 No. 8. (1994) 1437–44.

Akabayashi, A., et. al. "Galanin-Containing Neurons in the Paraventricular Nucleus: A Neurochemical Marker for Fat Ingestion and Body Weight Gain." *Proceedings of the National Academy of Sciences, USA.* Vol. 91, No. 22 (1994) 10375–9.

Alessio, H. M. "Exercise-Induced Oxidative Stress." *Medicine and Science in Sports and Exercise.* Vol. 25 (1993) 218–224.

American Psychiatric Association. *Diagnostic and Statistical Manual of Mental Disorders.* Fourth edition. Washington, D.C.: American Psychiatric Association (1994).

Anderson, G. H., & N. Hrboticky. "Approaches to Assessing the Dietary Component of the Diet - Behavior Connection." *Nutrition Reviews.* Vol. 44 (Suppl.) (1986) 42–50.

Anthony, Julie. "Psychologic Aspects of Exercise." *Clinics in Sports Medicine.* Vol. 10 (January 1991) 171–179.

"Aromatherapy: The Nose Knows?" *University of California at Berkeley Wellness Letter.* (May 1995) 4.

Ashley, D. V. M., et. al. "Breakfast Meal Composition Influences Plasma Tryptophan to Large Neutral Amino Acid Ratios of

Healthy Lean Young Men." *Journal of Neural Transmission.* Vol. 63 (1985) 271–283.

Austin, Elizabeth. "Diet-Pill Update." *Self.* (October 1995) 94–96.

Bancroft, J., et. al. "Food Craving, Mood and the Menstrual Cycle." *Psychological Medicine.* Vol. 18 (1988) 855–896.

Barone, Jeanine. "Five New Reasons to Get Physical." *Eating Well.* (July/August 1995) 26–32.

Benson, Herbert, and Eileen M. Stuart. *The Wellness Book.* New York: Birch Lane Press, 1992.

Berdanier, C. D. "The Many Faces of Stress." *Nutrition Today.* (March/April 1987) 12–17.

Bowen, D. J., and N. E. Grunberg. "Variations in Food Preference and Consumption Across the Menstrual Cycle." *Physiology & Behavior.* Vol. 47 (1990) 287–291.

Brzezinski, A. A., et. al. "D-fenfluramine Suppresses the Increased Calorie and Carbohydrate Intakes and Improves the Mood of Women with Premenstrual Depression." *Obstetrics & Gynecology.* Vol. 76 (1990) 296–301.

Byrne, A. and D. G. Byrne. "The Effect of Exercise on Depression, Anxiety, and Other Mood States: A Review." *Journal of Psychosomatic Research.* Vol. 17 (1993) 565–574.

"Can Your Mind Heal Your Body?" *Consumer Reports.* (February 1993) 108–115.

Caballero, B. "Brain Serotonin and Carbohydrate Craving in Obesity." *International Journal of Obesity.* Vol. 11 (Suppl. 3) 179–183.

Capuano, C. A., et. al. "Effect of Paraventricular Injection of Neuropeptide Y on Milk and Water Intake of Preweaning Rats." *Neuropeptides.* Vol. 24, No. 3 (1993) 177–82.

Carey, Benedict. "Overnight Sensation." *Health.* (September 1995) 36, 44.

Carroll, Doug. "Eating on the Road Turns into Battle of the Bulge." *USA Today.* (June 9, 1992) Section D.

Christensen, L. "Effects of Eating Behavior on Mood: A Review of the Literature." *International Journal of Eating Disorders.* Vol. 14 (1993) 173–183.

Christensen, L., and C. Redig. "Effect of Meal Composition on Mood. *Behavioral Neuroscience.* 107 (1993) 346–353.

"Clinical Aspects of Psychoneuroimmunology." *The Lancet.* Vol. 345 (January 1995) 183–184.

Cohen, S., Tyrrell, D. A., and A. P. Smith. "Psychological Stress and Susceptibility to the Common Cold." *New England Journal of Medicine.* Vol. 325 (1991) 606–656.

Coleman, Ellen. "Fat Burning and Exercise Dispelling and Misconceptions." *Scan's Pulse.* Vol. 14 (Spring 1995) 2, 3.

Cowley, Geoffrey. "Melatonin." *Newsweek.* (August 7, 1995) 46–49.

Craig, A. "Acute Effects of Meals on Perceptual and Cognitive Efficiency." *Nutrition Reviews.* Vol. 44 (Suppl.) (1986) 163–171.

Craig, A., and E. Richardson. "Effects of Experimental and Habitual Lunch-Size on Performance, Arousal, Hunger, and Mood." *International Archives of Occupational and Environmental Health.* Vol. 61 (1989) 313–319.

Cross, Audrey T., Bablez, D. and Cushmen, L. F. "Snacking Patterns Among 1,800 Adults." *Journal of the American Dietetic Association.* Vol. 94 (1994) 1398–1403.

Dalvit, S. P. "The Effect of the Menstrual Cycle on Patterns of Food Intake." *American Journal of Clinical Nutrition.* Vol. 34 (1981) 1811–1815.

Dalvit-McPhillips, S. P. "The Effect of the Human Menstrual Cycle on Nutrient Intake." *Physiology & Behavior.* Vol. 31 (1983) 209–212.

deCastro, J. M. "Circadian Rhythms of the Spontaneous Meal Pattern, Macronutrient Intake, and Mood of Humans." *Physiology & Behavior.* Vol. 40 (1987) 437–446.

"Deadly Depression." *Consumer Reports on Health.* (June 1995) 69.

DeBenedett, V. "Getting Fit for Life: Can Exercise Reduce Stress?" *The Physician and Sportsmedicine.* Vol. 16 (June 1988) 185–200.

"Does Exercise Boost Immunity?" *Consumer Reports on Health.* Vol. 7 (April 1995) 37–38.

Dollins, Andrew B., et al. "Effect of Inducing Nocturnal Serum Melatonin Concentrations in Daytime on Sleep, Mood, Body

Temperature, and Performance." *Proceeding of the National Academy of Sciences.* Vol. 91 (March 1994) 1824–1828.

Dreher. "Healing Journey." *Shape.* (1995) 54–56.

Drewnowski, A. "Changes in Mood After Carbohydrate Consumption." *American Journal of Clinical Nutrition.* Vol. 46 (1988) 703.

Drewnowski, A., et. al. "Food Preferences in Human Obesity: Carbohydrate Versus Fats." *Appetite.* Vol. 18 (1992) 207–221.

Drewnowski, A., et. al. "Taste Preferences in Human Obesity: Environmental and Familial Factors." *American Journal of Clinical Nutrition.* Vol. 54 (1991) 635–641.

Eller, Daryn. "Why We Crave Fat." *Walking.* (January/February 1994) 22–24.

"Emotions: How They Affect Your Body." *Discover.* (November 1984) 35.

"Empowering Older Women with Exercise." *Nutrition Updates.* (Spring 1995) 2–3.

"Exercise: A Little Helps a Lot." *Consumer Reports on Health.* (August 1994) 89.

Fernstrom, F. D. "Effects of the Diet on Brain Neurotransmitters." *Metabolism.* Vol. 26 (1977) 207–223.

Fernstrom. F. D. "Acute and Chronic Effects of Protein and Carbohydrate Ingestion on Brain Tryptophan Levels and Serotonin Syntheses." *Nutrition Reviews.* (1986) 44 (Suppl.) 25-36

Fernstrom, J. D. "Tryptophan, Serotonin and Carbohydrate Appetite: Will the Real Carbohydrate Craver Please Stand Up!" *Journal of Nutrition.* Vol. 118 (1988b) 1417–1419.

Fernstrom, John D., Ph.D. "Dietary Amino Acids and Brain Functions." *Journal of the American Dietetic Association.* Vol. 94 (1994) 71–77.

Fernstrom, M. H. and J. D. Fernstrom. "Brain Tryptophan Concentrations and Serotonin Synthesis Remain Responsive to Food Consumption after the Ingestion of Sequential Meals." *American Journal of Clinical Nutrition.* Vol. 61 (1995) 312–319.

Ganley, R. M. "Emotion and Eating in Obesity: A Review of the Literature." *International Journal of Eating Disorders.* Vol. 8 (1989) 343–361.

Garfinkel, D. "Improvement of Sleep Quality in Elderly People by Controlled-Release Melatonin." *Lancet.* Vol. 346 (1995) 541–544.

Goldberg, Carey. "The Simple Life Lures Refugees from Stress." *The New York Times.* (September 21, 1995) B1, B6.

Goldfarb, A. H. "Antioxidants: Role of Supplementation to Prevent Exercise-Induced Oxidative Stress." *Medicine and Science in Sports and Exercise.* Vol. 25, No. 2 (1993) 232–236.

Goodway, Jackie. "Exercise—The Stressor that Reduces Stress?" *Occupational Health.* (May 1987) 164–167.

Greeno, Catherine G., and Rena R. Wing. "Stress-Induced Eating." *Psychological Bulletin.* Vol. 115 (1994) 444–464.

Griffin, Kenneth W., et al. "Effects of Environmental Demands, Stress, and Mood on Health Practices." *Journal of Behavioral Medicine.* Vol. 16 (1993) 643–659.

Griffin, Katherine. "A Whiff of Things to Come." *Health.* Vol. 6 (Nov.–Dec. 1992) 34.

Groër, M. W., et. al. "Adolescent Stress and Coping: A Longitudinal Study." *Research in Nursing & Health.* Vol. 15 (1992) 209–217.

Halliwell, Barry. "Free Radicals, Antioxidants, and Human Disease: Curiosity, Cause, or Consequence?" *Lancet.* Vol. 344 (September 1994) 721–724.

Helsing, K. J., M. Szklo, and E. W. Comstock. "Mortality after Bereavement." *American Journal of Public Health.* Vol. 71 (1981) 802–809.

Holmes, S. "Stress and Nutrition." *Nursing Times.* (September 1984) 53–55.

"Home Exercise Equipment." *University of California at Berkeley Wellness Letter.* (December 1992) 4–5.

"Home Shopping Improvement." *Tufts University Diet and Nutrition Letter.* Vol. 13 (May 1995).

Irwin, Michael. "Stress-Induced Immune Suppression." *Annals of the New York Academy of Sciences.* Vol. 697 (1993) 203–217.

Irwin, Micheal, M.D., et al. "Partial Sleep Deprivation Reduces Natural Killer Cell Activity in Humans." *Psychosomatic Medicine.* Vol. 56 (1994) 493–498.

Jaret, Peter. "The Old Advice: Work Out. The New Advice: Walk the Dog and Take the Stairs." *Health.* (September 1994) 63–71.

Jenkins, R. R. and A. Goldfarb. "Introduction: Oxidant Stress, Aging, and Exercise." *Medicine and Science in Sports and Exercise.* Vol. 25, No. 2 (1993) 210–212.

Ji, L. L. "Antioxidant Enzyme Response to Exercise and Aging." *Medicine and Science in Sports and Exercise.* Vol. 25 (1993) 225–231.

Kanarek, R. B., and D. Swinney. "Effects of Food Snacks on Cognitive Performance in Male College Students." *Appetite.* Vol. 14 (1990) 15–27.

"Kitchen Notes." *Health.* (March/April 1993).

Kizilay, Patricia E. "Predictors of Depression in Women." *Women's Health.* Vol. 27 (December 1992) 983–987, 990–993.

Kopecki, D. O. "Controlling Stress in the Home and the Workplace." *American Association of Occupational Health Nurses Journal.* Vol. 34 (July 1986) 315–322.

Kratina, Karin. "Exercise Resistance." *Healthy Weight Journal.* (March/April 1995) 34–36.

Kusaka, Yukinori, et al. "Healthy Lifestyles Are Associated with Higher Natural Killer Cell Activity." *Preventive Medicine.* Vol. 21 (1992) 602–615.

Leatz, M. S. W., with M. W. Stolar. *Career Success/Personal Stress.* New York: McGraw-Hill, Inc., 1992.

Leibowitz, S. F., et. al. "Effects of Serotonin and the Serotonin Blocker Metergoline on Meal Patterns and Macronutrient Selection." *Pharmacol Biochem Behavior.* Vol. 45, No. 1 (1993) 185–94.

Lebowitz, S. F. "Specificity of Hypothalamic Peptides in the Control of Behavioral and Physiological Processes." *Annals of the New York Academy of Science.* Vol. 739 (1994) 12–35.

Lenfant, C., and N. Ernst. "Daily Dietary Fat and Total Food-Energy Intakes: Third National Health and Nutrition Examination Survey, 1988–91." *Morbidity and Mortality Weekly Report.* Vol. 43 (1994) 116–117.

Liebman, Bonnie. "E Is for Exercise." *Nutrition Action Healthletter.* (June 1995) 10.

Lieberman, H. R., et al. "The Behavioral Effect of Food Constituents: Strategies Used in Studies of Amino Acids, Protein, Carbohydrate, and Caffeine." *Nutrition Reviews.* Vol. 44 (Suppl.) (1986) 51–60.

Lieberman, H. R., et. al. "Changes in Mood After Carbohydrate Consumption Among Obese Individuals." *American Journal of Clinical Nutrition.* Vol. 44 (1986) 772–778.

"Lose Weight by Sniffing Fritos! Study's Findings a Tabloid's Dream." *Orlando Sentinel.* (October 17, 1992) Section D.

Maier, Steven F., et al. "Psychoneuroimmunology: The Interface between Behavior, Brain, and Immunity." *American Psychologist.* Vol. 49 (December 1994) 1004–1017.

Marano, Hara Estroff. "Chemistry and Craving." *Psychology Today.* (January/February 1993) 30–36, 74.

Margen, Sheldon, M.D., et al. "Nutrition for Optimal Health and Weight Control." *University of California at Berkeley Wellness Reports.* (1995) 32–34.

McCain, Nancy L., and Jonathan C. Smith. "Stress and Coping in the Context of Phychoneuroimmunology: A Holistic Framework for Nursing Practice and Research." *Archives of Psychiatric Nursing.* Vol. 8 (August 1994) 221–227.

McGrady, Angele, et al. "The Effects of Biofeedback-Assisted Relaxation on Cell-Mediated Immunity, Cortisol and White Blood Cell Count in Healthy Adult Subjects." *Journal of Behavioral Medicine.* Vol. 15 (1992) 343–354.

McLeod, Michael. "A Dose of Creativity." *Orlando Sentinel.* (October 15, 1995) Section D.

"Melatonin: Sleep Aid, Jet-Lag Antidote, Plus the Promise of More." *Environmental Nutrition.* Vol. 18 (November 1995) 6.

Messina, Mark, and Virginia Messina. "Healthy Rewards from Soy." *Veggie Life's Nourish.* Vol. 3 (December/January 1996) 1, 4.

Michaud, Claude, et al. "Effects of Breakfast Size on Short-Term Memory, Concentration, Mood, and Blood Glucose." *Journal of Adolescent Health.* Vol. 12 (1991) 53–57.

Monroe, S. M., et. al. "Onset of Depression and TIme to Treatment Entry: Roles of Life Stress." Journal of Consulting and Clinical Psychology. Vol. 59 (1991) 566–573.

"Mood Regulation." *American Psychological Association Journal.* (1994) 911.

Morrison, J. D. "Fatigue as a Presenting Complaint in Family Practice." *Journal of Family Practice.* Vol. 5 (1980) 795–801.

Nathan, Ronald G., et al. *The Doctor's Guide to Instant Stress Relief.* New York: G. P. Putnam's Sons, 1987.

Norton, Philippea, et al. "Physiologic Control of Food Intake by Neural and Chemical Mechanisms." Vol. 93 (April 1993) 450–454, 457.

Nowlan, Mary Hegarty, and Elizabeth Hiser. "The Hungry Mind." *Eating Well.* (May/June 1995) 28–34.

Nowlan, Mary Hegarty, and Elizabeth Hiser. "The Fat You Eat, the Risk You Take." *Eating Well.* (November/December 1994) 30–40.

"Older People Are Morning People." *Consumer Reports on Health.* (April 1994) 46.

Opstad, P. K. "Alterations in the Morning Plasma Levels of Hormones and the Endocrine Responses to Bicycle Exercise during Prolonged Strain. The Significance of Energy and Sleep Deprivation." *Acta Endo.* Vol. 25 (1991) 14–22.

Osterweis, M., F. Solomon, and F. Green. *Bereavement Reactions, Consequences, and Care.* Washington, D.C.: National Academy Press, 1984.

Pate, Russell, et al. "Physical Activity and Public Health." *Journal of the American Medical Association.* Vol. 273 (February 1, 1995) 402–407.

Patterson, R. E., et. al. "Low-Fat Diet Practices of Older Women: Prevalence and Implications For Dietary Assessment." *J. Am. Diet Assoc.* Vol. 96, No. 7 (1996) 670–9.

Pennington, Jean A. T. *Bowes and Church's Food Values of Portions Commonly Used.* 16th ed. New York: J. B. Lippincott Company, 1994.

"Physical Activity and Psychological Benefits." *The Physician and Sportsmedicine.* Vol. 20 (October 1992) 179–183.

Physicians' Desk Reference. 48th edition. Montvale, N.J.: Medical Economics Data Production Company, 1994.

Reaven, G. M. "Are Insulin Resistance and/or Compensatory Hyper-insulinemia Involved in the Etiology and Clinical Course of Patients with Hypertension?" *International Journal of Obesity and Related Metabolic Disorders.* Vol. 19 (Suppl.) (1995) 1, 2–5.

Reaven, G. M. "Are Triglycerides Important as a Risk Factor for Coronary Disease?" *Heart Dis. Stroke.* Vol. 2, No. 1 (1993) 44–8.

Reaven, G. M. "Effect of Metformin on Various Aspects of Glucose, Insulin and Lipid Metabolism in Patients with Non–Insulin-Dependent Diabetes Mellitus with Varying Degrees of Hyperglycemia." *Diabetes Metab. Rev.* Vol. 11, (Suppl.) (1995) 197–108.

Rejeski, W. J., et. al. "Acute Exercise: Buffering Psychosocial Stress Responses in Women." *Health Psychology.* Vol. 11 (1992) 355–362.

Rosch, P. J. "Exercise and Stress Reduction." *Comprehensive Therapy.* Vol. 11 (1985) 10–15.

Rossi, Ana M. and Charles A. Lubbers. "Stress at Work: Identification of Physiological Responses to Occupational Stressors." *American Association of Occupational Health Nursing Journal.* Vol. 37 (July 1989) 258–263.

Rossignol, A. M., and H. Bonnlander. "Prevalence and Severity of the Premenstrual Syndrome, Effects of Foods and Beverages That Are Sweet or High in Sugar Content." *Journal of Reproductive Medicine.* Vol. 36 (February 1991).

Selye, H. *Stress without Distress.* New York: New American Library, 1975.

Shaevitz, Morton, Ph.D. "Obesity: New Directions in Treatment." *Nutrition and the MD.* Vol. 21 (June 1995).

Silverstone, Trevor. "Appetite Suppressants: A Review." *Drugs.* Vol. 43 (1992) 820–836.

Slattery, M. L., et. al. "A Comparison of Two Methods to Ascertain Dietary Intake: The CARDIA Study." *Journal of Clinical Epidemiology.* Vol. 47, No. 7 (1994) 701–11.

Smith, A., et. al. "The Influence of Meal Composition on Post-Lunch Changes in Performance Efficiency and Mood." *Appetite.* Vol. 10 (1988) 195–203.

Smith, A., et. al. "Influences of Meal Size on Post-Lunch Changes in Performance Efficiency, Mood and Cardiovascular Function." *Appetite.* Vol. 16 (1991) 85–91.

Smith, Andrew, Anna Kendrick, and Andrea Maben. "Use and Effects of Food and Drinks in Relation to Daily Rhythms of Mood and Cognitive Performance. Effects of Caffeine, Lunch, and Alcohol on Human Performance, Mood, and Cardiovascular Function." *Proceedings of the Nutrition Society.* Vol. 51 (1992) 325–333.

Snyder, Barbara K., et al. "Stress and Psychosocial Factors: Effects on Primary Cellular Immune Response." *Journal of Behavioral Medicine.* Vol. 16 (1993) 143–158.

Somer, Elizabeth. *Food and Mood.* New York: Henry Holt and Company, 1995.

Spataro, J. A., and L. Van Horn. "Exercise to Reduce 'Potbelly.'" *Journal of the American Medical Association* (1995) Vol. 273, No. 6, 503.

Spring, B., et. al. "Carbohydrates, Tryptophan, and Behavior: A Methodological Review." *Psychological Bulletin.* Vol. 102, (1987) 234–256.

Spring, B., et. al. "Psychobiological Effects of Carbohydrates." *Journal of Clinical Psychiatry.* Vol. 50 (Suppl. 5) (1989) 27–33.

Spring, B., et. al. "Effects of Carbohydrates on Mood and Behavior." *Nutrition Reviews.* Vol. 44 (Suppl.) (1986) 51–70.

Stephens, Rebecca L., Ph.D., R.N. "Imagery: A Treatment for Nursing Student Anxiety." *Journal of Nursing Education.* Vol. 31 (December 1992) 314–319.

Su, H. Y, et. al. "Effects of Weight Loss on Blood Pressure and Insulin Resistance in Normotensive and Hypertensive Obese Individuals." *American Journal of Hypertension.* Vol. 8, No. 11 (1995) 1067–71.

Suchetka, Diane. "Is Laughter the Best Medicine? It's Certainly

Nothing to Sneeze At." *Orlando Sentinel.* (May 26, 1992) D-3.

Teich, Mark, and Pamela Weintraub. "Are Natural Cures a Prescription for Danger?" *Redbook.* (June 1995) 88–89, 111–114.

Tempel, D. L. and S. F. Leibowitz. "Adrenal Steroid Receptors: Interactions with Brain Neuropeptide Systems in Relation to Nutrient Intake and Metabolism." *Journal of Neuroendocrinoly* Vol. 6, No. 5 (1994) Oct. 479–501.

Tempel, D. L. and S. F. Leibowitz. "Glucocorticoid Receptors in PVN: Interactions with NE, NPY, and Gal in Relation to Feeding." *American Journal of Physiology.* Vol. 265, No. 5, Part 1 (1993) 794–800.

Tenebaum, G. "Physical Activity and Psychological Benefits." *The Physician and Sportsmedicine.* Vol. 20 (October 1992) 179–184.

Thayer, Robert E., et al. "Self-regulation of Mood: Strategies for Changing a Bad Mood, Raising Energy, and Reducing Tension." *Journal of Personality and Social Psychology.* Vol. 67 (1994) 910–925.

"The Stress-Resistant Person." *Harvard Medical School Health Letter.* (February 1989) 1–3.

"The Weighting Game." *Nutrition Action.* (May 1995) 4–7.

"The Stress in Your Life." *Health.* (October 1994) 46–47.

"Theories on Yo-Yo Dieting Unwind." *Tufts University Diet and Nutrition Letter.* Vol. 12 (December 1994).

Thoren, Peter, et al. "Endorphins and Exercise: Physiological Mechanisms and Clinical Implications." *Medicine and Science in Sports and Exercise.* Vol. 22 (1990) 417–428.

"Those Mighty Phytochemicals: Beyond the Benefits of Broccoli." *Environmental Nutrition.* Vol. 18 (November 1995) 1, 4.

"Vitamin E in the Diet." *Consumer Reports on Health.* (August 1995) 89.

Waterhouse, Debra. *Why Women Need Chocolate.* New York: Hyperion, 1995.

Watson, D., and J. W. Pennebaker. "Health Complaints, Stress, and Distress: Exploring the Central Role of Negative Affectivity." *Psychological Bulletin.* Vol. 96 (1989) 234–254.

"Weight, Fate, Set Point, Counterpoint." *University of California at Berkeley Wellness Letter.* Vol. 11 (June 1995) 1–2.

Weingarten, H. P., and D. Elston. "The Phenomenology of Food Cravings." *Appetite.* Vol. 15 (1990) 231–246.

"Which Exercise Is Best for You?" *Consumer Reports on Health.* Vol. 6 (April 1994) 37–38.

Williams, S. R. *Nutrition and Diet Therapy*, 6th ed. St. Louis Times Mirror/Mosby College Publishing, 1989.

Wurtman, J., et. al. "D-Fenfluramine Selectively Suppresses Carbohyrate Snacking by Obese Subjects." *International Journal of Eating Disorders.* Vol. 4 (1985) 89–99.

Wurtman, J., et. al. "Fenfluramine Suppresses Snack Intake Among Carbohydrate Cravers But Not Among Noncarbohydrate Cravers." *International Journal of Eating Disorders.* Vol. 6 (1987) 687–699.

Wurtman, J. J. "Carbohydrate Craving, Mood Changes, and Obesity." *Journal of Clinical Psychiatry.* Vol. 49 (Suppl.) (1989) 37–39.

Wurtman, R. J., et. al. "Carbohydrate Cravings, Obesity and Brain Serotonin." *Appetite.* Vol. 7 (Suppl.) (1986) 99–103.

Wurtman, R. J. and J. J. Wurtman. "Carbohydrates and Depression." *Scientific American.* (January 1989) 68–75.

Wurtman, Judith. *Managing Your Mind and Mood through Food.* New York: Harper and Row, 1986.

Wurtman, Judith J. "Depression and Weight Gain: The Serotonin Connection." *Journal of Affective Disorders.* Vol. 29 (1993) 183–192.

"Yoga: How to Stretch Away Stress." *Consumer Reports on Health.* (March 1995) 30–31.

Young, Simon N. "Some Effects of Dietary Components (Amino Acids, Carbohydrate, Folic Acid) on Brain Serotonin Synthesis, Mood, and Behavior." *Canadian Journal of Physiology and Pharmacology.* Vol. 69 (1991) 893–903.

Zwaan, Martina, and James E. Mitchell, "Opiate Antagonists and Eating Behavior in Humans: A Review." *The Journal of Clinical Pharmacology.* Vol. 21 (1992) 1060–1072.

INDEX